"I've battled the dragon of depression ever since I was in college, so I know firsthand how painful it can be. And because I've been a churchgoer since childhood, I also know how ill-equipped most churches are to help people survive it, much less fight it. *I Love Jesus, But I Want to Die* is a tender, practical guide for people of faith who struggle with depression. It weaves together vulnerable storytelling with simple practices to help you love yourself well, even when the dark cloud grows thick. Sarah Robinson has written a book I have needed for years. My only disappointment is that it didn't exist sooner."

—JONATHAN MERRITT, contributing writer for
The Atlantic and author of *Learning to Speak God from Scratch*

"This book is a beautiful heartbreak, a necessary look at the hard stuff we'd rather avoid talking about, and one we need now more than ever. For those struggling for a reason to keep going, and for those who love them, this is a must-read."

—JEFF GOINS, bestselling author of *The Art of Work*

"The way Sarah blends her personal story with helpful suggestions makes *I Love Jesus, But I Want to Die* an important read for anyone wanting to learn or understand more about the ways faith and suicidality can interact. Whether you're someone with similar experiences, a caring friend, or someone wanting to make your faith community safer for others, this book is for you."

—ROBERT VORE, therapist, co-host of the podcast *CXMH:
On Faith & Mental Health,* and human being
who has been suicidal while believing in Jesus

"In *I Love Jesus, But I Want to Die,* Sarah Robinson brings her hard-earned wisdom and the compassionate heart of a fellow traveler to the page. Sarah's words are a needed and helpful guide for folks who are navigating the difficult terrain of depression, trauma, and mental illness—while also looking for ways to experience Jesus in the midst of the storm. It's my privilege to highly recommend this important book."

—AUNDI KOLBER, licensed therapist and author of *Try Softer*

"In this book, Robinson places a candle in the middle of our darkness. By talking about the things Christians have too long kept hidden and hushed, she gives us room to hear our truest name: Beloved."

—K. J. RAMSEY, licensed professional counselor and author of *This Too Shall Last: Finding Grace When Suffering Lingers*

"There are excellent books about depression and suicidal thoughts, and even a few written by those with lived experience, but *I Love Jesus, But I Want to Die* is a one-of-a-kind book. Sarah Robinson opens to us the journal she kept during some of her worst days, giving the reader a tender glimpse of her intense struggles and suffering, as well as the beautiful hope she has found over time, without trying to tie a pretty bow around serious depression. This is a book to read for yourself or give to a struggling friend or loved one without the fear that depression and suicidal thoughts will be minimized, medicalized, or over-spiritualized. This is a really good book."

—KAY WARREN, cofounder of Saddleback Church

I LOVE
JESUS,
But I Want to Die

I LOVE
JESUS,

But I Want to Die

FINDING HOPE IN THE
DARKNESS OF DEPRESSION

SARAH J. ROBINSON

Foreword by Holly K. Oxhandler, PhD, LMSW

WATERBROOK

To Katie (and all those like her).
You've fought fiercely for wholeness and
turned your shattered pieces into something beautiful.
The world is better because you're still here.

Foreword

Dearest Reader,

I am so grateful for your presence in this precious moment and for your willingness to begin this book. Regardless of how this book has crossed your path, the pages ahead contain some of the most honest and tender reflections from one woman's journey navigating the intersection of faith and mental health.

Over the last several years, we've heard more courageous and heartbreaking stories surface alongside a growing amount of research that indicates our faith and mental health are interwoven in complex ways. As someone who has examined this intersection for more than a decade, I sense that these stories and studies are beginning to heal the complicated and unfortunately common divide between faith communities and mental health professions. Sarah's willingness to share her story and wisdom from lived experience helps us heal this division and empowers each of us to see these areas of our lives not as *either-or* but as *both-and*. We can have faith *and* struggle with mental illness, while moving toward our unique version of thriving.

Sarah and I connected a couple of years ago over our shared interest in this topic, and getting to know her compassionate spirit, gentle heart, and humble desire to care for others has been a gift. Her journey is unique, and yet the complex layers of what she's navigated echo what so many experience. For some, faith can be a powerful source of support, while for others, elements of faith can be part of the painful struggle. More often than not, however, it's a complicated combination of both.

Sarah's careful attention to the diversity of experiences you may bring to her story, her deep respect for both science and faith, and her humility merge into one of the most helpful books for understanding one person's lived experiences of mental illness who also loves Jesus with her whole heart.

This book is as much for those with mental health struggles perhaps wrestling with their faith as it is for many other groups. For example, the loved one who wants to better understand how to support their partner, friend, and/or family member working through symptoms of mental illness will be served in the pages ahead. Mental health care providers with clients who regularly mention the role of faith in coping with mental illness will find deeper insights into this intersection. Finally, faith leaders who recognize that mental health struggles are a current reality for one out of five of their community members' daily lives—and even more when factoring in loved ones who are impacted—will find helpful considerations ahead as they discern how to best serve their community.

I am deeply grateful for Sarah's courage, vulnerability, transparency, and tender care woven throughout this book. Even more, *I am deeply grateful for Sarah's presence in our world,* and I am honored by her willingness to share her heart with us. Sarah's life is a gift, and her story is one we can all grow from as we care for ourselves and for those around us.

Kindly,
Holly K. Oxhandler, PhD, LMSW

Contents

Author's Note

I know there might be times when you don't think you can go on. You don't have to face those moments alone. If you need immediate help or just someone to talk to when you feel overwhelmed, the National Suicide Prevention Lifeline is available 24/7 at 1-800-273-TALK (1-800-273-8255). For TTY users, use your preferred relay service or dial 711 then 1-800-273-8255. You can also reach the Crisis Text Line by texting the word HOME to 741741. Trained volunteers can help you navigate your situation, come up with a plan of action, and find your way back to a calm, safe place. Or call 911 or head to the emergency room—or an emergency mental health facility, if available in your area—if you can safely do so. You matter immensely and are worthy of support, care, and everything it takes to get better.

Introduction

HOW TO USE THIS BOOK

You're here because of the pain, aren't you? It might be a dull, gray ache that steals the color from your world or a raging inferno tucked just beneath your skin. If nothing else, it's persistent, sticking around long enough that you don't know if you can do this anymore.

I've felt that pain too. It's the stray dog I fed and couldn't get rid of, the colorless clouds, the oppressive fog. It's the weight on my chest, the rattle in my bones, the ghost that haunts the halls of my heart and mind and body. It's the curse I've carried like a scarlet letter, desperately wishing to be rid of it. And it's the disorientation of being plunged into midnight, finding myself terrified of the unseen things howling in the darkness. I'm sure there's something in that description that you can relate to; otherwise, you wouldn't be here.

If you don't personally know this agony, perhaps your heart is aching for somebody you care about: a loved one, a child or friend or spouse. Maybe a congregant or student. You're trying to understand his pain so you can offer some support, or maybe even help her find her way back to hope. It's a beautiful thing to want to lighten someone's load; thank you for loving well enough to learn about this illness.

Whether you're here for yourself or a loved one, I'm so sorry that you know this anguish. And I'm so glad you're here. Because there's something I've learned that I desperately want to share with you: it's possible to live a rich, beautiful life even under these heavy clouds.

This might sound absurd, especially for those of us who were taught that a life of faith means a life of victory, constantly overcoming the challenges in our paths. When healing doesn't happen, when our struggles remain, we're left wondering what's wrong with us for not experiencing this kind of triumph.

I've asked that question—*What's wrong with me?*—more times than I can count. But years of wrestling with depression, self-harm, and suicidal thoughts have taught me that sometimes the greater victory of faith is learning to walk with Jesus when suffering remains. This doesn't mean we're doomed to have miserable lives, controlled by mental illness. Instead, we can learn to live *well,* cultivate hope, and find new ways of experiencing the abundant life Jesus promised those who walk with him. This may not be the vision of what it means to thrive that we're familiar with, but it's no less valid.

Let me say it again, friend: you are not disqualified from the abundant life Christ promised to all his followers. There is beauty, hope, and even joy ahead for you; you aren't too fractured to experience it. There's a richer relationship with the God who loves you and never leaves you. There are wonderful surprises, and there's freedom you can't yet imagine, *even if* you don't experience complete healing from mental illness in this life.[1]

I know this because these promises—of hope even *in* the dark, of joy coexisting *with* sorrow—are etched throughout Scripture, from beginning to end. Science is constantly revealing ways we can live more whole and more healthy lives, even with depression. I'm confident of this, not just because I read about it in the Bible or in a scientific research study, but because I'm living it.

I've had lifelong depression and anxiety. Over the years, I've attempted suicide and used self-harm to cope with the pain. Even now, I still have hard days and weeks. But in spite of all that, my life is marked by genuine peace and even joy because I've learned how to care well for myself, I've realized what God *really* thinks and feels about me and my struggles, and I've found how I can support my brain and body to experience more joy and contentment. Now when hard days come, I know I can ride the waves of depression without drowning under them. That's what this book is all about.

This book won't cure you. It won't fix everything for you (believe me, I wish it could). But it can help you find a path to a rich, fulfilling life despite living with severe depression.

I want you to know that I am not a mapmaker. I can't plot your journey in perfect detail, showing you every milestone and landmark on the way to a life you want to wake up to, even on your hardest days. I am simply a fellow traveler, perhaps a few paces ahead on the journey, able to turn back and share some of my steps and missteps. I've picked up some information that can help make your way easier, and I hope to help you avoid some pitfalls and navigate well. But mostly I want to give you hope.

I am not a therapist, doctor, or scientist. I am a bit of a nerd who loves to understand how things work and why. In this book, you'll find research, tips, and tricks that have helped me to care for myself and find healthy rhythms in the midst of my depression. However, I cannot give medical or psychological advice, so please don't take what I share in these pages as a replacement for working with well-trained, licensed professionals. In fact, if you don't already have a solid team around you, that's the first thing I would suggest. Skip ahead to the chapters on working with doctors and therapists if you need some help navigating the process to find a good one.

I'm also not a trained theologian. You won't find a systematic explanation of the theology of sickness and suffering here. Yes, I'm a former youth pastor, but the majority of my theological understanding has come from personal study, listening to people who believe differently than me, and the experience of walking with God in hard places.

In these pages, you'll discover the things I wish I had known when I began my journey of integrating my faith and mental health—the tools I wish I had much earlier. Sometimes that means I'll talk about the spiritual side, focusing on ways to pray or things I've learned about the love of God. Other times, I'll dig into the practical and scientific side by sharing the work of professionals who have discovered how we can work with our brains and bodies to live well, even in the fog. When it comes to the research, I'll leave the nuances to the experts—just think of these parts as an introduction to the voices I've learned a great deal from. If something piques your interest or seems particularly relevant to your experience, please follow up with additional reading. There are plenty of resources in the notes and appendix B to check out.

How to Use This Book

I wish I could sit with you at a coffee shop, hear your story, and share the bits and pieces of my journey that would most encourage you. Of course, since I can't sit down with everybody, some parts of this book will be more immediately relevant than others. That's okay.

You'll find the chapters arranged more or less chronologically according to my experience, but feel free to skip around based on what seems most helpful to you. Each chapter focuses on a lesson I learned along the way: from becoming a new Christian, to discovering that loving Jesus didn't take away the darkness of depression, to the process that taught me to cultivate hope even in my worst seasons. Some chapters will be practical, offering specific steps to take or exercises to try. Others deal more with mindsets, beliefs, and emotional challenges that we often experience on our mental health journeys.

One Thing You Need

When you've been wrestling despair for a long time, it starts to feel impossible that anything will ever change. That loss of hope for a better future is a dangerous place to be. And for somebody who deals with severe depression and suicidal thoughts, a complete loss of hope can be life threatening.

For many years, I believed that I was stuck in my anguish unless God chose to heal me from the depression and anxiety that plagued me. I lived in fear of the next depressive episode that would send me into a pit so deep I wasn't sure I'd ever climb out. It was a brutal time. What I didn't know is that I wasn't at the mercy of my circumstances.

Eventually, I discovered a crucial truth about thriving: it's not about being healthy or ill. It's about having a set of learnable skills that I can develop and apply to any circumstance. Dr. Carol Dweck, a professor from Stanford, has spent her career researching the way our beliefs change our ability to thrive. She discovered that a simple change in mindset makes all the difference.

The first perspective is the one I had about mental health for most of my life. It's called a fixed mindset, and it assumes that our abilities and traits are predetermined and unchangeable. That means we believe that some people are naturally smarter, or better at math, or able to cope with hard things, while others missed out on those abilities. When we have a fixed mindset, we believe that setbacks and failures reveal who we really are and will always be.

The second perspective is one that has changed my life. It's called a growth mindset because the core belief is that we can learn and change our abilities and traits. Sure, some people might have more natural talent at art or basketball, but anybody can learn to be a better artist or basketball player through practice and education. With the growth mindset, failures and setbacks don't have anything to say about who we are as people; they just reveal areas in which we can grow and learn.[2]

In Dr. Dweck's research, she found that mindset makes a huge difference in people with depression. Patients with a fixed mindset experience more severe depression, more tormenting thoughts about themselves, and more disruption to their lives than those with a growth mindset. They aren't able to keep up with their work or care for themselves. In fact, Dr. Dweck explained that "this mindset seems to rob [patients] of their coping resources."[3]

Those who have the growth mindset still ache with the pain of depression, still struggle to get out of bed and face another day. But they also believe that they can get better and that their choices make a difference in their lives. "The worse they felt, the more motivated they became and the more they confronted the problems that faced them," Dr. Dweck said.[4] In other words, the simple belief that things can change—that *we* can change—can make a world of difference in whether we're able to keep going in the darkness.

A growth mindset sounds a lot like hope, doesn't it?

That doesn't mean you're going to be able to change your whole life in an instant, and it certainly does not mean you can simply think your way out of your illness. Instead, this perspective—that thriving is possible—helps us pursue things that make a huge difference, such as prayer, medication, therapy, and good self-care.

A Note on Difficult Content (Trigger/Content Warnings)

It's a delicate balance when writing about depression, suicide, and self-harm. On one hand, it can be incredibly validating to hear someone talk about the things you haven't been able to voice. We all want to know we aren't alone and that somebody else gets it. On the other hand, reading about self-harm or a suicide attempt can stir up dark thoughts and urges that make you feel overwhelmed and unsafe. We call this being triggered, and it's a physiological reaction to something especially distressing. It commonly happens as part of a trauma response, but we can also experience triggers with other mental health challenges (such as a struggle with an eating disorder or suicidal thoughts). Being triggered doesn't mean you're weak. It's just your body's way of saying it doesn't feel safe and it's looking for a way to cope with an overwhelming experience.

With all this in mind, I've attempted to err on the side of caution in what I share, but it's important for you to skip sections that don't feel safe for you. While everyone experiences different triggers, I've highlighted some particularly difficult sections to make them easier for you to skip. If you do notice yourself feeling distressed (anxious, short of breath, lightheaded, numb, or having more thoughts of hurting yourself), that's a sign you should take a few deep breaths, skip the section, or set the book down for a bit. It is much more important for you to stay safe than it is to read every word in this book.

A Note on God and Faith

I haven't always known God to be loving, compassionate, and close. I didn't believe God loved me for the first five years of my faith because painful circumstances, complicated church experiences, and trauma made it hard for me to connect with the God I had always heard is kind and gracious. You might relate to that struggle, my friend. If, like me, you've been angry with God or haven't always felt he could be trusted, that's okay. If you've struggled with faith or aren't even sure what you believe, you are welcome here.

In these pages, you'll see how I've come to know a God who is present in the dark and refuses to bail on us. I speak of God as relentlessly kind, knowing that we who wrestle with mental illness desperately need to know divine comfort and grace. God is love (1 John 4:8), after all, and there is immense healing in knowing that love is real and for us, even during our worst moments.

It's been my joy to connect with readers from many different streams within the Christian faith, with traditions as beautiful and varied as the body of Christ. This is precious to me because God is greater than all our boxes and we need each other to reveal more and more of God to the world. But it's also precious because the kindness of God is not bound to any denomination, worldview, or political perspective—and neither are mental health challenges.

Most of us with mental illness have experienced trauma of some type,[5] so we bring those experiences to bear on our perceptions of God. For example, it can be difficult to see God as a good parent if we've only ever experienced toxic parenting. For that reason, and many others, assigning a gender to the God who created both male and female as equal image bearers is uncomfortable for many.[6] That said, I've chosen to speak about God in traditional ways, including using masculine pronouns, though I acknowledge that may be difficult for believers with different backgrounds and faith experiences. I've done this because it is most familiar to the majority of my readers as well as me. If this is foreign or strange to you, please keep in mind that all our little words are simply signposts pointing to a God whose fullness defies description.

When It Feels Too Hard

I've lived with mental illness long enough to know there will probably be times when the clouds feel like they're closing in and you're not sure you can face the day. We're going to talk about some things in this book that won't be easy to do, some changes that will take practice to implement. And there might be moments when you grow impatient with the slow pace of change or don't think you have it in you.

Take courage, my friend.

The mindset research I mentioned earlier is exciting because it proves that we really can change our lives. But what's even better than that is the fact that we, as believers, have the additional strength and support of God to help us. By the time the apostle Paul wrote about learning to navigate hardship, he had endured severe trauma: beatings, imprisonment, and even starvation. He was near the end of his life, writing from a prison cell, when he said, "I can do everything through Christ, who gives me strength" (Philippians 4:13, NLT).

The same God who raised Jesus from the dead, who empowered Paul through such suffering, is with us now. Throughout this book, we'll see over and over how God is with us to help us in the darkness. We don't just have the God-given ability to renew our minds (though we'll look at the science behind brain change and what this means for us). We have Christ himself, present in our lives through his Spirit, to strengthen us in our weakest, darkest moments.

When those moments come, take courage. When you don't feel hopeful, remind yourself of this truth: you can learn to live well despite mental illness. And whether depression becomes a distant memory for you someday or it remains part of your life as it does for mine, you are not disqualified from the rich, abundant life that Jesus promised. There are good things ahead, my friend. And you are worth whatever it takes to get there.

Part One

DYING

One

Loving Jesus Doesn't Cure You

TRIGGER/CONTENT WARNING—The first section of this chapter discusses a suicide attempt. If you are currently struggling with thoughts of suicide or self-harm or believe reading about a suicide attempt would be unhealthy for you for any reason, please skip the gray highlighted section. Remember, if you notice any distress as you read, take a few deep breaths, step away, and distract yourself with pleasant thoughts or activities before returning to the book. Take good care of yourself.

I was a Christian the first time I tried to kill myself.

I'd contemplated suicide countless times over the years, emptying a bottle of pills into my hand to feel their weight or fantasizing about stepping in front of a car. The thoughts were constant, vicious, and unspoken. But I never made an actual attempt until eight months after committing my life to Christ in a tiny warehouse church.

I'd done all the "right" things. I got baptized, went to church every time the doors were open, swapped my old friends for relationships with youth-group kids, read my Bible, prayed, and worshipped. I'd gone to conferences and even on my first mission trip. And with my charismatic, miracle-focused church, I'd preached the gospel and prayed for people to be healed on the streets of our city.

I was convinced I should have felt better.

But I didn't.

Instead, the hope of my new faith faded into a gnawing sense of disappointment. Why did I still hurt so much? Why wouldn't God fix me? Everyone at my new church seemed to receive constant reassurances of God's love and approval, but he seemed bitterly silent to me. It only reinforced the raging self-hatred I'd carried for so long. *God doesn't even want me. It's my fault; I'm too selfish and sinful. It's never going to get better.* I felt sick all the time and everything seemed so hollow. I was sure I was doomed to an unending ache and I couldn't bear it.

So, one late-spring evening when my house was empty, I found myself sitting on the kitchen floor, pressing a knife into my eager skin. There was no note, no explanation, just a blade and some blood between me and relief from the bone-crushing suffering.

At first I felt calm, resigned. That hollow nausea was still in my chest, but at least I didn't have to live with it much longer. I took a deep breath, bracing for the pain. But then I froze statue-still. My heart pounded and I started to sweat as I seemed to wrestle a force outside myself. I willed myself to press in just a little more, just enough, but I couldn't do it. I couldn't make it happen.

Finally, I relented. I flung the knife across the room.

"You won," I spat in God's direction, flushed with anger. It was all his fault I couldn't be free from the pain.

I don't know how long I sat on the dirty kitchen floor, but I eventually realized I didn't want my family to find me there, so I got up and put the knife away. I climbed into bed, put on a worship CD, cursed God, and went to sleep.

I told only one person about the attempt, a kid in my youth group who was like a big brother to me. I don't know if he ever told anybody else, if he thought I was being dramatic, if he really understood what I was saying. And I don't remember his response. But I do know he never mentioned it again. My secret struggle with the darkness remained a secret.

As an adult, I look back with compassion on those around me; they were as clueless about how to handle mental illness as I was. What was that seventeen-year-old boy in the early 2000s supposed to know about suicide prevention? What were my twenty-three-year-old youth pastors in a "name it and claim it" church supposed to tell me when I talked about how much I was hurting?

It's not that they didn't do their best to lead and love me well; they just didn't have the tools they needed to care for someone with severe depression. Chris and Jenny were newlyweds just figuring out what it meant to be married, work, go to college, and run a youth group all at the same time. To be in ministry—especially in a small church—is to live under a microscope, and as neither had any formal training, they depended on the theology they picked up from the culture around them. To say they were stretched thin would be a massive understatement, but they had big hearts and longed to make a difference in the lives of others.

A few months after the attempt, when I hesitantly shared bits of my pain, they carved time out of their impossible schedules to invite me over for dinner at their four-hundred-square-foot apartment. Chris talked to me about overcoming lies with Scripture and spending more time in the presence of God, while Jenny made me a card covered in glittery stickers and Bible verses about freedom, overcoming the flesh, and having the mind of Christ. They prayed with me and encouraged me to praise the Lord, especially when I didn't feel like it.

That night, I left their cramped apartment with a jumble of emotions. My youth pastors did everything they knew how to do, and their love for me was obvious. But I also felt frustrated because my experience didn't match the promises, confused because I didn't understand why. Regardless, I received the same message they had from our church culture: Jesus fixes everything. We just have to co-operate.

When I began to self-harm in college, Chris and Jenny would say they'd found out I had started cutting "again," as though it had been something that plagued me in the years before I came to faith. I never corrected them, never told them how I only started carving my pain in my skin after I pledged my life to Christ.

I understood the unwritten rules: This isn't the story I'm supposed to tell. This isn't how it works for "good Christians." You meet Jesus and then everything gets better. You discover you're loved and find your purpose in Christ, and you're filled with unspeakable joy. Life is good, God blesses you, and you're too busy serving others and worshipping God to hurt like that. That's how it's supposed to work.

You don't find yourself slipping deeper beneath the waves, drowning while surrounded by people who can't even see the water. You don't starve in the middle of the elaborate feast set before you. You don't watch the light grow dim and wonder how everyone else around you is able to see anything at all.

But that's what happened to me.

Looking back, it's not tough to see how my church—and countless others—came to believe that loving Jesus cures all ills. We loved a good testimony, proof of God working in our midst. Week after week, people would stand up and share how they were healed, delivered, or rescued from some difficult thing or another. The message was clear: Jesus fixes broken things. Jesus works miracles.

Our senior pastor was a firm believer in the miraculous and leaned heavily on verses that talk about God healing anyone and everyone. We were taught that God promised perfect health when he brought the Israelites out of Egypt and that these verses were just as applicable to us:

> He said, "If you will listen carefully to the voice of the LORD your God and do what is right in his sight, obeying his commands and keeping all his decrees, then I will not make you suffer any of the diseases I sent on the Egyptians; for *I am the LORD who heals you.* (Exodus 15:26, NLT)

> And the LORD will protect you from all sickness. *He will not let you suffer* from the terrible diseases you knew in Egypt, but he will inflict them on all your enemies! (Deuteronomy 7:15, NLT)

We recited Psalm 103:3 together every Sunday to build our faith: "He forgives *all* my sins and heals *all* my diseases" (NLT). And Isaiah 54:17 promised that "no weapon formed against you shall prosper" (NKJV).

It wasn't just the Old Testament that promised God would heal and restore everything. Luke 4:40 recorded that when sick people were brought to Jesus, "no matter what their diseases were, the touch of his hand healed *every one*" (NLT). And Matthew 7:11 clearly showed that if we asked our Father for good gifts, he would give them to us.

Isn't the crux of Christianity that there is a good God who loves us and paid the price for our sin and suffering? Isn't his character full of kindness and compassion? Doesn't it make sense that his will is always to heal us?

That theology sounds true and beautiful—and it fits well with the very human desire to avoid suffering. In my church, I believe this was taught from an innocent desire to see God glorified and impact the lives of his children. It was never intended to cause harm or undermine the full truth of the gospel. But it's woefully incomplete, ignoring the many times in Scripture that God—for whatever reason—allowed people to endure sickness and suffering without swooping in to rescue them from it.

Like countless other churches, my community glossed over verses that talked about suffering as part of life or times when God allowed painful situations to remain. It wasn't until years later that I saw a fuller picture of suffering in Scripture. I found this truth woven throughout the New Testament, in verses that get little notice: God doesn't always heal people.

In Galatians 4:13–14, we learn that Paul was sick when he came to Galatia—sick enough that it would have tempted the people to reject him. Instead, they took him in and cared for him. Later, we learn that one of Paul's companions was left behind to rest because he was sick (2 Timothy 4:20). He wasn't healed to go on with the important missionary work.

Even Jesus didn't always heal everybody. There's this beautiful story in John 5 in which Jesus comes up to a pool called Bethesda in Jerusalem. It's surrounded by crowds of people in desperate need of healing. They're paralyzed, sick, or blind, waiting for the moment when the water starts to bubble and stir. They believed that the bubbling was actually caused by an angel and whoever could get into the pool first would be healed.

So Jesus comes up, makes his way through the crowd, and stops in front of a man who had been sick for almost forty years. "Do you want to be healed?" he asks.

This poor, sick man doesn't know who Jesus is, doesn't know his life is about to change, and just says he can't get into the water in time. If you've read the story, you know what happens next: Jesus tells this man who has been ill for thirty-eight years to get up—and he's healed instantly.

It's a beautiful story for so many reasons: the way Jesus saw somebody who wasn't even looking for him, the way the grace of God made way for healing, and the heady possibility that one encounter with the Lord can change everything—but we usually miss one important fact.

There were crowds of people Jesus didn't heal that day.

Tons of them. In fact, the King James Version calls it a "multitude." And Jesus just made his way past them, maybe even stepping over them as they lay on mats and cobblestones around the pool.

Why do we ignore this?

I think it's because we're afraid.

Maybe we're afraid we'll be stepped over, passed by, or ignored by Jesus.

Maybe we're afraid that God isn't really as good as we want to believe, and it's hard to hold the tension of a Father who both gives good gifts and allows us to endure suffering.

We have to wonder what it means if God is able to heal but doesn't heal us. God may be good, but is he good to us when our anguish seems to go unnoticed by an all-powerful, all-loving being? Is there something horribly wrong with us that keeps us from experiencing his kindness and grace?

It's scary when we recognize God's goodness in the lives of others but not our own. And in some church structures, those anxieties can be reinforced by those in the pulpit or the pews. You may even have experienced the kind of toxic leadership that uses those fears as a tool for control or selfish gain, telling you God will bless you only if you give more money or conform to certain expectations. But in most churches, this plays out less as a desire for control and more as a longing for security.[1]

This subtle prosperity-gospel faith teaches us that if we do the right things—whether it's having enough faith, giving financially, or working hard enough—God will bless us. Maybe we don't expect him to reward us with a fancy car or big bank account but surely with happiness and healing and answers to our problems. On some level, we are convinced that the circumstances of our lives are evidence of how happy he is with us. We may labor in prayer or performance, but our ultimate goal is to be good enough to please God. This belief system is especially dangerous because it teaches people struggling with mental illness that our circumstances are our own fault. That searing shame drives some of us to despondency, denial, or even resignation. Others, like me, are driven to furious activity, trying desperately to crack the code that will lead to our healing.

So we keep showing up at church, desperately going through the motions of our Christian duty, but hope slips from our grasp week by week. We give and pray and serve, but nothing seems to change.

In the midst of a culture that celebrates victory, we start to believe God is good—just not to us. God is present, but not with us. God is gracious, but not to us. Those thoughts feed a cancerous self-hate, reinforcing the lie that our sickness is beyond God's reach.

When I'm drowning in the darkness, aching with indescribable pain, I don't need to hear that if I just pray or read my Bible or become a better Christian, God will heal me.

I need to know, deep in my bones, that loving Jesus doesn't cure me. I need to know that being a Christian doesn't automatically make me better and that it's not supposed to.

This may sound discouraging, but I think it's actually good news: being a Christian doesn't guarantee we won't struggle. In fact, Jesus actually *promised* that we would struggle. He gave us a heads-up about this in John 16:33. Before going to the cross, during his final hours with the disciples, Jesus said, "In this world you will have trouble" (NIV). The NLT says "you will have many trials and sorrows."

Ouch, Jesus. We don't want trials and sorrows. I sure don't. If I'm honest, part of me wishes for the simplicity of a transactional, vending-machine faith: put in the right payment in the form of good-Christian behavior, receive the right reward in the form of health, wealth, and happiness.

But here's why it's good news: it means nothing is wrong with us when we struggle in the darkness. It means we haven't failed, we aren't bad Christians, and we're not lacking faith. Jesus promised we would have trials and sorrows and hard times.

And here's the even better news: Jesus has overcome the world.

That's the other half of John 16:33: "Take heart, because I have overcome the world" (NLT).

In my darkest moments, when shame gripped me and kept me bound, I didn't need to hear that God had promised to heal me. I needed to hear God was with me, that there was nothing wrong with me, and that God was no less present in my pain than in the triumphs of others. I needed to know that Christ, who has overcome the whole world and all its suffering, wouldn't leave me alone in mine.

We need faith that makes room for suffering, that refuses to deny the brokenness of this sin-sick world and our place in it. We need theology that honors the ache while clasping tightly to the hand of a God who refuses to abandon us. We need a community that doesn't wait for Jesus to wave a magic wand and fix us before they can accept us.

Sweet friend, there is nothing wrong with you. You are not a bad Christian for toiling under the crushing weight of depression. Mental illness is not a failure of faith or evidence of a flimsy prayer life. It's simply a common part of the human condition, one that many people will experience.

The brokenness in our world shows up in a million shattered ways: sickness and trauma, betrayal and grief. Some of us suffer because of biology, coming from a family with a long line of mental illness. Others live with the fallout of harmful choices others made. And many endure the heavy waves of grief that are sure to come with great loss.

Jesus came to earth in the midst of this suffering. He was surrounded by it constantly. And, yes, there were certainly times when Jesus performed miracles, when he touched and healed the brokenness. And each time revealed something rich and beautiful about God: that he cares immensely about us, that he is powerful, and that he is near.

But there were many, many times Jesus simply gave hope for the future. And that hope reveals the same things about God's care, power, and presence with us. Hope is no less powerful than miraculous healing. It still shows us that he is near and he cares deeply.

Because the truth we forget when we read short Bible stories is this: every person healed by Jesus went on to suffer in countless ways. Each still lost loved ones, still lived in the wreckage of a world that desperately needs to be made right.

My friend, we are not alone in the aching dark. We walk with saints who have gone before us—a great cloud of witnesses who intimately know sorrow and heartache and grief.

And we are not missing anything. There's no enigma to unravel, no right combination of behavior and prayers, no secret decoder ring that holds the answers to escape or deliverance.

Those who have gone before us know a truth we sorely need: there are some things about God that can be experienced only in affliction. When we endure suffering, including mental illness, we have the opportunity to know God in an incarnational way.

I get it. When you're shaking so hard you can barely breathe and you think your heart might literally explode, you're not so sure you want to know God like that. But I've learned there is no better way to know the Comforter than by being comforted. There's no peace like what you experience in the fire of anxiety.

Maybe it's really hard to make this mental shift right now. That's okay. Sometimes it's more difficult to sit in the darkness and believe God is with us there than it is to cling to a prosperity-gospel faith that promises healing if you do the right things.

It's okay if this is hard and doesn't make sense. It's okay if you're angry and can't understand why God would allow this pain. It's okay if you're struggling to move past the fear that God is good to everyone except you. We'll dig into more practical ways to find wholeness later in the book, but I want you to know that this is a journey, and wherever you are right now is okay.

Still, in the midst of the ache, cling to this truth: There is nothing wrong with you. You have nothing to be ashamed of. And even in the darkest night, there is hope.

Two

People Say Terrible Things
(But We Still Need Them)

I don't know why I said yes. I was supposed to be out partying with friends. I was not supposed to be sweltering in a tiny warehouse church on a Friday night.

I thought I was a Christian, that just claiming the name and sending up an occasional prayer was enough. I didn't have a clue about following Jesus, about surrender and repentance and trust.

I'd never been to a youth group and had rarely gone to church. When a kid I'd just met in my high school yearbook class invited me to go hang out with a bunch of strangers in a warehouse on a Friday night, I took him up on it without having much of an idea of what to expect.

Before that night, I was depressed and suicidal. In fact, I don't remember a time before the consuming ache, before I just wanted to stop hurting. In elementary school, I often stared out the school bus window, imagining getting hit by a semitruck or climbing out the back as we barreled down the highway. I longed to go to sleep and never wake up, but every morning dawned relentlessly. So each day, I'd get up and head to school, go through the motions, pull straight As, and never let anybody see the monster gnawing on my insides.

As I got older, weekends became exhausting. I spent them pretending to be okay, playing the role I'd carved out for myself in my friendship circle. By high school, I was a consummate caretaker, holding a friend's hair back when she threw up from drinking too much or comforting another after a fight with a boyfriend or girlfriend. I'd busy myself cleaning up when the party was over, collecting red cups and empty food wrappers.

I drank and danced with them, tried smoking pot, tried coming up with the stupid, reckless ideas that sound fun when you're a teen, but none of it ever helped me feel better. I'd always felt out of place around my peers, like a piece to the wrong puzzle that wouldn't quite fit no matter how close it looked. I laughed and smiled so not even my closest friends would know how often I wished for death. It was as if a pane of glass separated me from the rest of the world, from whatever it meant to be normal. By the end of the summer before my sophomore year, I was so bone weary of pretending to have fun that I'd retreat to a dark corner when nobody was looking, venting my pain in grim poetry.

Maybe it was just a change in routine that sounded appealing the first Friday night of that school year. Maybe it was the fact that I wouldn't have a role I needed to fill, that I wouldn't have to pretend as much. Whatever it was, I found myself surrounded by high school and college students. Everyone was shockingly friendly as I milled around and navigated the awkwardness of new relationships. I recognized a handful of people from school, but most were new to me. I didn't know it then, but I was meeting some of my dearest lifelong friends. And my life was about to change.

I'd been to church a handful of times, so I expected a familiar music-announcements-sermon format. But this was different. There was no message, no altar call, no invitation to repentance that night. Instead, I watched as people around me raised their arms and closed their eyes, belting out the words to each song.

Ashley, a girl I recognized from school, grabbed the microphone and talked about how God saw each of us as precious jewels, sparkling rubies and sapphires and emeralds. Her voice broke as she described a fierce, jealous love, and tears pooled in the corners of her eyes. Jenny, in an '80s raglan T-shirt and bouncy, blond ponytail, made her way around the room, praying for students scattered through the front of the sanctuary. I sat on the floor at the end of the first row, my heart jumping into my throat as she knelt next to me. I was nervous, unsure of what to expect. She gently placed her hand on my shoulder and prayed for me as the band continued to play through a terrible sound system. I don't remember what she said, but I drew my knees to my chest and sobbed while the words of the song washed over me.

Even now, when I read Psalm 84, I'm transported to that night and I hear my friend Michelle singing in her plaintive voice a now-familiar chorus from "Better Is One Day" by Matt Redman:

> Better is one day in Your courts
> Than thousands elsewhere

Somewhere between Jenny's prayer and Michelle's singing, my chest started to burn. I didn't have words for what was happening, why I was crying, or why my heart felt that way. But that night, I left knowing I wanted to go back, to experience more of whatever it was.

The words from that song haunted me for weeks. I began to believe them—that this strange thing I had experienced was the presence of God. That it wasn't just better than anything else but was the answer to everything. When Michelle sang those words, they rattled something inside me: Maybe the heaviness and longing I'd always felt was hunger for this God. Maybe my heart and flesh had been yearning to be close to him. Maybe that's what this was all about—and maybe, maybe, if I listened to those words and spent all my time close to him, I would stop hurting. The empty, aching void would be filled, and I would find what it means to really live.

That's the story we were supposed to tell as Christians, I quickly learned.

But that wouldn't be my story.

Weeks stretched into months as I threw my entire being into my faith. I lived and breathed for it, showing up at church every time the door was open, helping distribute food in the community after services, setting up chairs, and eventually joining the worship and prayer teams. In the heady days after I became a Christian, I was so eager to please God. But I was perhaps just as eager to please my pastors and my new Christian friends. I desperately wanted to belong. I craved the validation of my church community, to know I was on the right path. That I was enough.

As months went on and the enthusiastic honeymoon period of my faith wore off, I made a sickening realization: that gaping void was still lodged between my ribs. I didn't understand what was going on inside me—after all, loving Jesus was supposed to make it all better. In my confusion and shame, I frantically sifted through possible explanations. It had to be a spiritual problem, the darkness of my own sin and selfishness.

In hindsight, I know that it was simply my undiagnosed, untreated mental illness that made it feel impossible for me to "choose joy" and experience the "abundant life" that was supposed to be mine in Christ. In a church culture that valued victorious testimonies and taught that taking antidepressants was a sign of a lack of faith, it seemed obvious to me that my struggles were the result of some hidden sin or failure as a believer.

That belief was only reinforced when I hesitantly began to talk about my pain with believers around me. I shared some of my angst-ridden poetry with a friend from youth group; she nervously giggled, saying "That scares me," and changed the subject. I tried to figure out why I felt shut out from the joy others seemed to experience—I didn't feel any sense of purpose, so maybe I hadn't discerned my calling yet? Perhaps God had me in a "spiritual desert" to help me mature? Or maybe God just didn't like me and refused to speak to me the way everyone at church seemed to hear from him. As I considered these possibilities, I asked pastors and ministry leaders for prayer. But the results didn't line up with our expectations. We believed the power of God was present in our lives to do the miraculous, to provide all our needs, and bless us. We emphasized God's omnipotence and verses that talked about anything supernatural: healing, multiplying loaves and fishes, walking on water, and casting out demons. But when people prayed for God to speak to me, to break off the spirit of oppression, and to restore the joy the Enemy had stolen, nothing happened. I was still hurting and confused, ashamed that I couldn't be the joyful Christian I believed I should be.

At the same time, I was learning that honestly talking about the ache and confusion inside was seen as a barrier to victory. We also emphasized verses like Proverbs 18:21 that talked about the power of our words. If "death and life are in the power of the tongue," and God brought creation into existence with nothing more than a few words, then our words mattered immensely. From the pulpit and the pews, I constantly heard that making a "negative confession" could prevent us from receiving the healing and blessings God had for us. The words we spoke, coupled with faith, could essentially create our lives; instead of saying, "I'm catching a cold," people said, "I'm catching a healing." We had to be positive; if we weren't, we could inadvertently curse ourselves or those around us. This meant it was difficult to speak openly of depression—or any heartache—when my community was used to speaking of blessings even in the midst of deep pain.

People liked to quote those old sayings, the ones that sound vaguely spiritual and true enough to pass for genuine comfort:

- "Choose joy."
- "God doesn't give us more than we can handle."
- "Just focus on other people and serve more. Don't be selfish."
- "There's something wrong if thinking about Jesus dying for you doesn't make you happy."
- "Don't make mountains out of molehills."
- "If you can't say anything nice, don't say anything at all—even about yourself."
- "Thoughts of self-harm are clearly demonic."
- "Where's your faith?"
- "Don't be so overly dramatic."

There were others, sometimes more subtle, and terrible things people said to and about others experiencing pain and grief:

- "If you had more faith, your child wouldn't have died."
- "You must have some hidden sin."

- "She's making it up or exaggerating. She's not really abused."
- "God does everything for a reason."

But the one I hated the most was "this too shall pass." Sometimes I thought I would punch somebody in the face if she said that to me.

I get it. It's meant to be reassuring, especially when it's coming from somebody with a few more years under his belt. It's meant to remind us that life is full of ups and downs, that things change. The hard circumstances we're experiencing now won't last forever. "The sun'll come up tomorrow" and all that. I know this phrase is helpful to some, and I've even adopted a version of this phrase ("dark days don't last forever") that I whisper to my own heart when I'm afraid a depressive episode will never end.

But throwing out a platitude—any platitude—is incredibly dismissive. It's gut wrenching to have our experiences and pain so quickly belittled, invalidated, and tossed aside. It also misses something important when we're talking about the most serious challenges in life: sometimes, they *don't* just pass. The grief of losing a loved one may eventually lose some of its initial fury, but it won't fully disappear. Sometimes, broken relationships aren't mended. And there are many ailments, including mental illnesses, that don't just pass.

For some people, seasons of depression are as fleeting as summer storms; they're fierce and frightening but gone quickly. And many of us with clinical depression will experience what are known as depressive episodes, in which symptoms flare and things get hard for a while. Those episodes may pass. But they might not. Some people experience chronically low moods that go on for years if left untreated. Some people get caught in the cycles of bipolar disorder, moving from dangerous highs to crushing lows over and over. Some people have illnesses that are even harder for the untrained layperson to understand, like schizophrenia and borderline personality disorder—things that don't just pass on their own.

In my life, depression hasn't passed. Sure, the major depressive episodes come and go. I recognize the cycles now, and it *is* comforting to remind myself that my lowest moments don't last forever. There will come a day when I feel better again. But clichés like "this too shall pass" and "choose joy" don't speak to the crushing reality of mental illness.

———

I need you to understand something: the people who said some of these hurtful things to me were wonderful. They were church moms who stuffed me full of delicious home cooking and held me when I cried, ministry leaders who prayed for me constantly, and young pastors who made time to mentor me when I was stubborn and cynical. They loved me well and supported me in more ways than I could count.

These were the people I called when I had a flat tire or a blinding migraine and couldn't drive myself home. A handful of families scraped together the funds to buy me an old car so I could move out, go to college, and get a job when I graduated from high school. I sat at their kitchen tables and learned to do my taxes, study the Bible, and speak up when there's something I'm scared to say. They taught me how to worship and pray and help others connect with God.

They saw good things inside me, called out purpose and destiny, told me I was a leader and could influence others in a positive way. They provided scholarships and helped me raise money to go to youth conferences and on mission trips that I could never have afforded on my own.

So much of who I am today is because of the loving influence of this community of faith. I needed them. Especially in the depths of my depression, I needed them. They may have said some hurtful things to me, but they also hugged me, had me over for dinner, and trusted me with their children. They may have caused pain, but their genuine love for me gave me hope time and again when I was ready to end my life. One couple had me stay with them when I finally admitted I was suicidal. My church became family to me, and many of us are close to this day.

Here's what I've learned: people are broken and I can be certain they will, at times, fail me. Sometimes people do things that are without excuse, and there are definitely people out there who have been toxic and harmful. In those situations, it's important to set boundaries, distance yourself, and find safer people to open up to. But most people aren't like that, even when they say terrible things. The vast majority of the time, they just don't know better. They're ill equipped, or they're scared to say the wrong thing, even though they genuinely want to help. (Note: If that's you, check appendix A in the back for simple ways to talk to those who are struggling.)

Sometimes, I've just had wrong expectations. In this chapter, I've talked about what it was like to be a young, new believer in a church that wasn't equipped to deal with my mental health challenges. There were certainly things that could have been done better, and my heart aches for my younger self from those days.

But I also ache for all the volunteer ministry leaders who had very little training and impossible expectations placed upon them. I imagine how fast their hearts were beating as they tried to say the right things, how they stayed up way too late preparing messages when they had to get up early for their day jobs, how they may have wrestled under their own pain without receiving the support they needed.

My friend, as I invite you to hold the tension that people can both care for and wound us deeply, I'm not trying to excuse or minimize difficult experiences at the hands of other believers. Even if the pain was caused inadvertently, it is still valid. It's not okay when Christians shame each other for taking medication or blame very natural struggles with mental health on spiritual problems.

The distance of time allows me to see the love and care as well as the hurt, to recognize that most relationships incorporate both. Still, you may not have experienced a supportive and loving church family; if that's the case, I am so sorry. Maybe you've been betrayed by trusted friends and it seems to have cast a shadow over all believers. Perhaps trauma, anxiety, or neurodiversity (differences in the ways we learn and think) make it tough for you to try again. Please know it's okay and normal that this feels so hard. Even with having people who loved me well, I feared ever opening up about my mental health and traumatic experiences.

Still, we need people. We need the mixed bag of blessing and brokenness that is humanity.

We simply cannot thrive without other people. But we can learn to find safe, supportive community to walk with us in our hard seasons. And that's God's desire for us.

Made for Relationship

From the first moments of mankind, we were made for relationship. Adam had hardly gotten the hang of breathing before God recognized he wouldn't thrive alone (Genesis 2:18). In *The Anatomy of the Soul,* after detailing the neurological processes that cause us to bond to each other, Curt Thompson, MD, tells us that "being connected [is] as natural and as necessary as breathing. . . . God, with his hands having been deep in the mud into which he exhaled life, senses the man's lack of completion, declaring, 'It is not good for the man to be alone.'"[1]

I love that picture of God up to his elbows in the dirt of creation, seeing that his precious creation needed something more. That something was relationship, not just with God himself, but also with other people. Thompson went on to say that this need to connect with others, this "attachment has been kneaded into the most primitive fibers of our being."[2]

We need each other.

It can be difficult to hold the tension between needing a safe place to open up and understanding that none of us responds perfectly all the time. That struggle isn't unique to our generation. In the Bible, well-meaning friends thought they could help people struggling with grief, depression, and thoughts of suicide with simple explanations or platitudes.

We see this in the book of Job, particularly in the "miserable comforters" (Job 16:2) who said some awful things to Job. But even these friends were able to honor the first seven days of sitting shiva in silence with him, entering into his grief (Job 2:11–13). In this Judaic tradition that's still practiced today, friends and family come to sit quietly with the person grieving, not speaking unless the bereaved speaks first. But for Job, things went downhill after a while when his friends stopped sharing his pain and instead tried to explain the horrible things that had happened to him.

They tried to speak for God, telling Job he must have sinned or otherwise brought the calamity upon himself. They had believed that somebody could experience such loss and hardship only if he had sinned. But God turns that belief upside down. At the end of the book, God shows up and essentially tells Job's friends they don't know what they're talking about, that they spoke foolishly. Job's friends believed they were helping, but they only caused him more pain and misrepresented God in the process (Job 42:7–9).

Healed in Relationship

Annie Rogers wrote, "What has been wounded in a relationship must be, after all, healed in a relationship."[3] We all intuitively know that life is better when we have a support system. Loneliness is painful and absolutely makes depression worse, so it makes sense that being surrounded by a supportive community helps us survive depressive episodes. Studies have shown that people who experience a challenge in life, like unemployment, are much less likely to develop mental health problems if they have a healthy network of friends and family. Social support has also been proved to help victims of bullying manage anxiety better. One study even found that strong community literally helped people stay alive.[4]

But the evidence isn't just for social support in general; believe it or not, research has linked involvement in religious services (i.e., church attendance) to lower depression symptoms.[5] It also shows that communities like churches provide the kind of positive social support we desperately need to live well despite mental illness.[6]

Making sure our support systems include people in our faith communities can make us more likely to move past depressive episodes, less likely to relapse, less likely to give in to suicidal impulses, and more likely to feel a sense of happiness and well-being.[7] In other words, we can stack the deck in our favor by getting involved in healthy, supportive churches.

Finding Healthy Community

So how do you find a healthy support system? Here are some practical tips on how to find a safe, healthy community:

If you're not involved in a church right now, there are a few clues to watch for as you look for the right community for you. Social media, podcast episodes, or prior sermons on YouTube can be great resources. It might take some digging, but if you find topics on mental health that are encouraging, hopeful, and nonjudgmental, it's a good bet that it's a safe place for you. Visit an online service if you can. Is the church compassionate and kind? Do the leaders and members offer dignity and honor to those they talk about? Do they protect and serve the vulnerable?

Do leaders seem to display humility? Are they ready and willing to refer people out beyond the four walls of the church? Churches that talk about us all being broken and messy and imperfect—especially when the leaders talk about their own brokenness, doubts, and failures—are often more comfortable walking with people through hard things.

Of course, you can always reach out via email or social media and ask a few questions. Does the church keep a list of licensed mental health professionals for referrals? Are there support groups available, such as Celebrate Recovery, Fresh Hope, or Grace Alliance groups? Sometimes more resources are available in larger churches, but it can be difficult to find connection. This is tough when you're depressed—and don't have energy or drive. And when you're anxious, it can be flat out terrifying to walk into a new group, especially if you deal with social anxiety. But if you do find a larger church that feels like a good fit for you, it's absolutely worth it to gather your reserves to find a small group within it for closer community.

Be open to a different denomination or "stream" of faith. Don't sacrifice essential beliefs, but it's okay to be flexible on things that really aren't central to the faith. One of my friends who was raised in southern charismatic churches has found an incredible Episcopal community that feels like home and family to him. There's something beautiful about experiencing a different flavor of faith and learning about our brothers and sisters who practice differently than we are accustomed to. Maybe you are used to strict, expository teaching and a rigorous "holiness" focus. It is not a compromise to check out a church with a more contemplative style of worship, topical preaching, or greater emphasis on grace. The body of Christ is vibrant and diverse, with each tradition highlighting different aspects of the character of God—and sometimes, dipping a toe into another stream can be just what we need.

As I mentioned above, small groups are incredible for making a large church feel smaller—but they can be intimidating, especially when we're struggling. Try anyway. Be brave and share a little bit of your struggle (in future chapters we'll explore how to do that). Sometimes people won't understand, and some might try to respond with answers. That's okay. Try again. More likely than not, others in the group have dealt with something difficult and will be able to relate. Watch for how the group responds when other members share hard things; it's a good indicator of how they'll respond to you sharing your pain.

We Need Them Anyway

Here's what I know: People are broken and messy and imperfect. They fail me time and time again. They will never be enough to fill the broken places in me, never enough to mend my soul.

And I need them anyway.

It's a beautiful mystery: *People* can't heal me, not of themselves. But so often, when God bends low to restore my soul, he does it through the same broken people. I've swung wide on a pendulum from desperately looking for humans to heal me, to shutting down and building walls to keep everyone out. Neither works very well. But in the middle, I'm finding balance. I'm finding that I can look only to God to transform me, and he wants to use the people he's placed in my life to do it.

Three

"I'm Not Disappointed in You"

TRIGGER/CONTENT WARNING—This chapter discusses self-harm. If you are currently struggling with thoughts of suicide or self-harm or believe reading about self-harm would be unhealthy for you for any reason, please skip the gray highlighted sections. Remember, if you notice any distress as you read, take a few deep breaths, step away, and distract yourself with pleasant thoughts or activities before returning to the book. Take good care of yourself.

When I started cutting, the shame drove me to it. I'd feel it burning in my skin with sickening intensity, and I didn't know what to do. I didn't know how to soothe it.

For several years after my first suicide attempt, I kept moving, kept the plates spinning, kept taking on more responsibility and leadership at church. I was trying so hard to be good, but somewhere along the way, this belief that I was intrinsically toxic had taken root. It colored all my perceptions. I'd believed serving others would get my mind off myself, that knowing I had purpose would help, so I'd thrown myself into everything I could: work, college, worship practice, mentoring high school students, countless hours helping at church.

Hard as I tried, I couldn't outrun the pain or find the sense of purpose I was looking for. So shame followed me around like an old stray dog I'd fed. I didn't understand then that shame is a self-reinforcing loop, turning back on itself to create more and more as we feel shame about our shame.

It reached a crescendo in college when I was trying to juggle far too many responsibilities but found myself drowning under waves of depression, grief, and unresolved trauma. Of course, I didn't know that's what was going on; I hadn't yet spoken to a doctor or therapist. As far as I was concerned, it was a spiritual problem, and I had been walking with the Lord long enough that I should have been better. *Certainly, I should be over this by now.*

But I wasn't over it. I wasn't able to hold all the pieces together anymore, and I couldn't figure out how to get rid of the indescribable feeling of badness inside me. Like there was something terribly wrong with me, and I had to let it out.

The year had grown harder, week by week and month by month. There were days I couldn't scrape together the energy to get out of bed. There were brain-splitting migraines, and when I saw my doctor, she asked about stress. But I didn't understand my emotions well enough to recognize it—I genuinely thought I was handling the pressure just fine.

Of course, I wasn't handling it just fine; by spring of my sophomore year, I was falling behind. On the days I managed to peel myself out of bed and stumble out the door, I either spent classes staring out the window in a fog of hazy numbness or sobbing in my car. It became apparent I was going to fail most of my classes—I, the straight A student to whom school always came so easily. I couldn't bear the thought of Fs on my transcript, so I dropped every course I could without penalty. My Spanish teacher wouldn't let me drop her class, but her eyes were kind as I sat in her office. I barely made it through the verbal final without crying.

Anxiety roiled my stomach, making it impossible to eat. I lost twenty pounds and people started asking if I had an eating disorder. It seems strange now that I never entertained the thought that this might be depression. I didn't have words for the pain or know how to process my thoughts and feelings in healthy ways. I just knew I was sinking and felt so alone. Eventually, I couldn't even cry, couldn't talk about it with anybody.

Instead, I wrote it in my skin like a dirty, terrifying secret. I despised myself for it, but it was the only way I could let off some of the pressure. The burning sense of badness built up in my chest, and I had to release it somehow. It doesn't make sense if you haven't been there, but the sight of the blood felt like purging some of that pain. The evidence of hideous failures spiderwebbed across my skin, but I kept them hidden. I had to.

I remember being so afraid that somebody would find out that I found myself anxiously tugging at hemlines to cover the wounds. Others may have thought it was for modesty's sake, but I knew better. Still, even greater than my embarrassment and fear of others finding out was the sense that I was failing and rejecting God. As I read through my old journals from the summer I was cutting, I read things like *I'm not just empty—I've become a vacuum, taking on more and more in the absence of your presence.*

I believed that my struggle with self-harm removed me from the presence of God. Like when I did this thing to cope, God couldn't be close to me anymore. I saw it as sin—something that divides and distances us from God, even if we already belong to him.

For far too long, the crippling shame kept me silent. But then I found myself standing unannounced on some friends' porch on a hot July night. Their kids were long in bed. I was twenty and terrified, and I didn't think I could dig my voice out of the hollow of my chest. I swore they could hear my pounding heart. Every passing moment felt like time was stalling, both never ending and like I was about to die. And the truth is, I wanted to.

That night, the high desert air was hot and still, void of humidity. I had parked my car in front of an open field, stars and silvery-blue moonlight coloring my pale skin and a steel blade. I just wanted to stop hurting. I realized that if I didn't get help, I was going to die. For the first time, I knew I wasn't in control. That scared me enough that I was finally ready to ask for help.

I could think of only one place to go, so I put away the blade, pulled a bandage from the first-aid kit, and tended to the cuts. I hesitated, my hand on the keys in the ignition, staring into the blue night. They'd known I was struggling, had seen my broken pieces before. But nothing like this. Nothing so humiliating.

I turned the key, started my car, and went down the back roads at a crawl. Between the field and their house, I must have pulled over half a dozen times, choking on fear and desperately gathering any remaining courage. I was shaking when I pulled into their driveway, unsteady on my feet as I stepped out of my car. Their front door was open to let in the cool night breeze. I tried to swallow the lump growing in my throat and stepped inside.

I walked into their house with a tight, grim smile, painfully conscious of the bandages under my clothes. They stared, wide eyed, from the couch as I sat in the rocking chair across from them, hugging a pillow to my chest. When they asked what was wrong, I could barely voice the ugly words: I had been cutting and wanted to die. I felt like I was about to vomit.

They were quiet for a moment, and I couldn't stop trembling in the long pause. Angela said I should stay with them for a while; I knew she wasn't asking, but telling me. Then, Michael spoke words I didn't know would change my life:

"I'm not disappointed in you."

It rattled me. I was speechless.

"I don't think less of you."

09/02/07

Lord I'm struggling. I need Your help. This week has been really rough— I've been sad + lonely + angry at numb. I've cut myself and beated myself, wished for the end, tried so hard to hide it.

I'm not just empty—I've become a vacuum, taking on more and more in the absence of your presence. I've tried all sorts of things to cope, but in my own "strength" they all fail. I'm frustrated because I don't know what to do, if there's some switch I'm just not flipping, or if there's anything I can do to get free.

I'm having a really hard time, Lord. I don't understand why things have not changed inside of me after all these years. Most days I've forgotten how to fight. I've believed that there is no hope of a better life, a healed mind + whole heart. I feel like a failure, a lost cause, and that belief is so sticky.

Will you help me? Be my hero, my rescue, my deliverer. Please. Please just be with me. Don't lose me, God, please don't let me be lost.

How can this be? How?!? I was horrified, as though they were excusing something unpardonable, something foul. *A near college dropout, a youth leader harboring this secret, and you're not disappointed? How could you look at me with compassion after this?!?*

But they were honest words, and though I was incredulous, they stuck. They resonated in my soul, echoing loud as the first words I heard that pushed past my shame. Those words started a new phase in the war inside me.

The climb out of that dark episode was slow and agonizing, with failures and relapses along the way. I now know this is the path of recovery—stumbling forward and falling down—though I didn't recognize it then. There were times when I felt wild and caged, looking for escape as I spent long nights on their couch and long days going through the motions of reading books to their kids and trying to press myself into some mold of normal. But those simple words of acceptance still rolled around inside me, gave me hope, and kept me going. They shaped me and became part of me.

Eventually, I would learn healthier ways of caring for my hurt, to understand depression and self-care and love. But in that season, the grace and compassion I received from people (and a lot more from Jesus) made hope grow inside me. I learned that even though I hated it when people told me *this too shall pass,* it's true that dark days don't last forever and that better days do come again. But even if they do last forever, I'm not alone in the darkness. I began to treasure small moments of joy, to document moments of grace and gratitude even when I made my bed in the depths of hell.

Nothing to Hide

When we're caught in destructive patterns or simply fighting to survive, it's easy to think that God is surprised or caught off guard by our thoughts and actions. We believe God is disappointed, angry, or even downright disgusted by our actions.

Most of us have something that we're ashamed of: eating disorders, addictions, sexual behavior, broken relationships. Some of us feel like we've done things that God can't or won't forgive. Some of us have experienced abuse that left deep marks, telling us it's our fault that we weren't loved well or protected. All of us sometimes feel like we're not good enough in one area or another. Any of these things can trigger deep shame.

Shame is not our birthright. The kind of shame that keeps us silent and separated was never part of the plan. We might believe that we're just living under Eden's curse, when humanity lost the ability to be naked and unashamed in the presence of one another and of God (Genesis 2:25). That's where humanity learned to cover not just our bodies, but our souls, trying to piece together fig leaves and to hide from God in the bushes (Genesis 3:7–10).

But listen to the echoes of a brokenhearted Father: *Where are you? Who told you that you were naked?* Even after Adam and Eve messed up, God didn't want them to hide in shame. He still wanted them to come close to him, to bring their brokenness to him.

When Michael said he wasn't disappointed in me, I felt rattled, disoriented. But as those words worked their way into my soul, I came to a slow realization. If these are the honest words of one person's imperfect love, can anything ever make God disappointed in me? I believed I was utterly pathetic when I showed up that night, but Michael and Angela's love could handle me even then. Did that mean the familiar refrain from Romans 8:39 that nothing in all creation can separate us from the love of God could be something real and alive to me?

If I truly believe in the omniscient, loving God revealed through Jesus Christ, I believe in a God who cannot be surprised. Psalm 139:1–4 paints a picture of God knowing every part of our lives:

> O Lord, you have searched me and known me!
> You know when I sit down and when I rise up;
>   you discern my thoughts from afar.
> You search out my path and my lying down
>   and are acquainted with all my ways.
> Even before a word is on my tongue,
>   behold, O Lord, you know it altogether.

The God who knows our words before they come to mind, who is intimately acquainted with all our ways, can never be disappointed in us because we cannot surprise him. Disappointment comes from not experiencing an expected outcome, and God doesn't anticipate us to behave in ways he already knows we're not going to. He expects us to fall down, to make mistakes, to struggle, and to even sin sometimes because he already knows our frailties. He may grieve and ache over our struggles and choices, but he wants us to just come to him with our pain and problems.

This is the God illustrated in the story of the prodigal, the father who ran to the son who had rejected and dishonored him. In a culture where it would have been unthinkable for a son to ask for his inheritance while his father was living, much less squander it and then come back to his father's house, the father ran to embrace his son. When the rest of the world would have expected the son to be rejected at best (and possibly executed for dishonoring the family), the father was too eager to celebrate the return to even let the son finish his apology (Luke 15:11–32).

This father, with his reckless acceptance and lavish love, is a picture of the very God who draws near to us in our pain, compassionately present in the battles we face. This is the God of whom Isaiah said, "The LORD longs to be gracious to you" (Isaiah 30:18, NIV). This is not a God who wants us to hide from him in shame. Instead, Scripture is clear that Jesus is compassionate and sympathetic to our circumstances and that we are to come to him boldly for the grace and help we need (Hebrews 4:15–16).

There is no failure that can't be forgiven, no weakness God doesn't have grace for. There is nothing we can hide from him. We don't need to be ashamed of our brokenness before God. He is already intimately acquainted with all our ways; there's nothing to hide.

The Science of Shame

It's hard to explain why I started self-harming, beyond the fact that the shame drove me to it. But shame also kept me silent for too long, terrified to open up about the darkness and to get the help I needed. That's why it's such a deadly tool in depression's arsenal. It doesn't have to be this way; shame doesn't have to control us. But first, it can be helpful to understand just what is going on inside us when we feel this crushing emotion.

Dr. Curt Thompson defined shame as "a felt sensation of deep inadequacy" or of there being something wrong with you. He says the neural circuits are a self-reinforcing loop, which means we often feel shame for feeling shame. We all experience shame, even children as young as eighteen months old, Thompson suggested—though, of course, they're far too young to understand why. When we experience this profound sense of inadequacy at a young age, especially without loving support to help us navigate it, we are left with a toxic "residue of shame" that is easily reactivated later in life.[1]

This experience is common for children whose parents don't consistently meet the child's physical or emotional needs. If the child internalizes this experience, she will eventually grow to believe she is intrinsically bad, inadequate, or shameful. In a strange way, that belief provides a sense of stability and security: if the people who are supposed to love and care for us aren't able to do that well, it's less scary to believe there's something wrong with *us* than to believe that our caretakers are unreliable and can't provide what we need.[2]

We don't need to experience serious neglect or abuse to be vulnerable to shame; we all experience it from an early age, and we all are vulnerable to reactivating the patterns of shame in our minds when we experience anything similar to what initially created the patterns. Because mental illness isn't often discussed in many social circles and can make us feel like we're not good enough, it seems like an easy way for those patterns to get triggered in our brains.

And we don't just feel the physical sensations of shame, the sickening weight and desire to disappear. We tell ourselves stories about our struggles with the darkness: *I should be better by now. I should just get over this. I should be more grateful because other people have it worse than me.* Aundi Kolber, a licensed therapist, observed, "People *love* to criticize emotions." Instead of responding compassionately to our feelings, Kolber said, we try to either disconnect from them or shame ourselves for them.[3]

That's how shame keeps us silent: it's a dangerous feedback loop that keeps us from speaking up, reaching out, and reconnecting. But the important thing to recognize is that the *feeling* of something being deeply wrong with us isn't a reflection of reality. For most of us, the shame loop started when we were quite small, when someone didn't respond well to our needs. This is crucial to remember because it means that feeling of shame is lying to us. It's not an accurate reflection of who we are.

What Now?

Shame is a compulsive liar. We must accept that the toxic, destructive messages it gives us are untrue before we can resist the instructions it gives. But once we know it's lying to us, that there's nothing wrong with us, we can do what it takes to get better.

That doesn't mean the *feeling* of shame will disappear right away or that you won't struggle with it anymore. I so wish that were true. Some days, I still feel the burning sensations in my skin and the sickening sense of not-enoughness that used to drive me to self-harm. Now, instead of obeying those urges, I remember that shame isn't the boss of me, and I give voice to the struggles, both in my relationship with God and with the safe, loving people in my life.

Right now, fighting shame may look like sharing a little piece of your struggle with somebody who cares about you. It might look like making an appointment with a doctor or therapist, or asking around for a recommendation for a mental health professional. Or maybe it's imagining somebody else in your shoes—someone who is fighting mental illness, wrestling with unfair circumstances, or just trying to stay afloat—and thinking about what you would say to him. Think about the kind of compassion you'd extend to him. Then, extend that same compassion to yourself.

Extending compassion to myself has become a lot easier as I've had the immense privilege of being entrusted with the tender, broken places others have invited me into. There have been times when others have come to me with their own shame, even their own struggles with self-harm. Whenever possible, I try to give the gift of those same words I received so long ago:

"I'm not disappointed."

"I don't think less of you."

"You're not a failure."

"You're still worth loving."

I know how reassuring these words can be when you've been trying so hard but keep failing.

I don't know your struggle or your story. But if we were together, talking over coffee, and I saw your eyes lower as you confessed the things you wish you could overcome, I'd say, "I'm not disappointed. I don't think less of you." I'd tell you I've been there too, that I've felt the sting of self-hate for all I couldn't change. I'd tell you I carry the scars of that burning shame in my skin even now. I'd pray that ultimately you'd hear the voice of Jesus reshaping the shame into security. I'd hope the words rattle around inside until you know nothing can ever separate you from his love.

But we can't all meet over coffee, and I can't look you in the eyes and tell you that. So, my friend, tell yourself. I hope you find the courage to talk to people and are met with grace and mercy. But if you're not there yet, tell yourself. Extend to yourself the grace that you need to hear. Tell yourself things like, *I'm not disappointed in you, and neither is God. You have nothing to be ashamed of. You're not a bad person for struggling, and you deserve help. You're worth whatever it takes to get better.*

I want you to hear these words in the depth of your soul. I may not be the person you most long to hear them from, but what matters most is that they are the words God is speaking over you. He cannot possibly be surprised by your actions. He cannot possibly be disappointed in you. There is not a moment he wishes you were something different than you are. You are exactly, deeply, utterly beloved. He is not disappointed in you.

Four

Learning to Be Loved

I was a Christian for five years before I believed God *really* loved me. My faith was born in a community that emphasized intercession, and I came to believe that *true* prayer was a fevered thing, full of passion and vigor. If it wasn't loud and active, it wasn't true prayer. A friend once joked that he didn't get why it was called "quiet time" if people were supposed to be praying.

We often invoked the verse that says "the effectual fervent prayer of a righteous man availeth much" (James 5:16, KJV). Somehow, that sounded to me like the results of prayer had more to do with passion, intensity, and the quality of my faith than the God who is able to answer. So my prayers were often fevered, begging things, supposing God would hear and respond if I was passionate and asked enough times. More often than not, those desperate prayers disintegrated into frantic pleading: *Please, just make me better. Make me good enough. Why won't you fix me? I know you can. Why don't you just wave that magic wand you have somewhere up there and make me better?*

When these pleas weren't answered, I grew bitter and angry. I became furious that God had abandoned me to so much pain. It felt like he was refusing to help. More than once, I screamed and swore at him, saying I wished he would show his face so I could slap it.

On the surface, I was angry at God because I believed I couldn't live up to his impossible standards for constantly joyful believers. But it was just a thin veil stretched over the truth: my core belief was that I was wretched, toxic, and unlovable, even to God himself. I was certain I was a nuisance to God, just barely tolerated.

Of course, I knew the right things to say: *God loves everyone. Everyone includes me.* But if I was completely honest, I thought God *had* to love everyone. *It's not like he* wants *me or even* likes *me. He doesn't have a choice in the matter.* Besides, if I was broken and shameful beyond repair, why would God want me?

My friends Michael and Angela called me out on those beliefs the night I showed up on their doorstep. They saw the searing self-hate and named it. It surprised me, almost as much as it had when Michael had said he wasn't disappointed in me. I'd never considered how much I hated myself, how much I believed I wasn't worth taking up space in the world. I'd never stepped outside my own thoughts or considered that they were anything but objective reality, the absolute truth about me.

Although Michael and Angela didn't know to name it as depression or trauma, they knew one thing needed to change. "You need a genuine experience with the love of God," Angela told me. "We need to start praying for that."

My voice was small when I responded, just a weak, "Okay." I didn't quite buy it, that the solution could be so simple after so many years of unanswered prayers. But I was desperate, and my friends were in it with me, so I was game to try. I started praying. *God, help me experience your love in a way I can't deny.*

It didn't happen the way I expected nor as soon as I'd hoped. For months, it seemed my prayer went unanswered; there were many wild, desperate nights when I didn't think I would make it. There were more times I coped with the pain by wounding myself, more planned suicide attempts when I was convinced I couldn't hang on any longer. But somehow, little bits of hope kept me going. I showed up at church one Sunday, fresh cuts hidden under my clothes, and went up for prayer.

My pastor, who now knew I was struggling with self-harm, took my hands, looked me in the eyes, and said, "You're doing such a good job," before praying for me. I shook my head and tried to swallow my sobs, convinced of how badly I was failing. Still, bits of encouragement like that kept me going as I continued to pray for an experience with the love of God, never realizing the compassion and care of those around me *was* the love of God.

It was a long, hard season, one when I scarcely dared to believe that my prayers could come true. I endured more than I hoped, borrowing strength from those who believed better things for my future. I couldn't see the love of God through my friends because I was still looking for a big, magic-wand moment when everything would change forever. I wanted a line in the sand that I could step over and know I was never going back.

Months after Angela and I started praying, I got a letter in the mail. I'd been awarded a scholarship to study abroad in Paris. It didn't make any sense; I'd sent my application late and it was weeks past the deadline for notifications. Nevertheless, I was accepted and found myself on a plane to a country where I didn't speak the language or know a single person.

When I arrived, it didn't take long before I realized that my host mom—who I'd been told would speak English—only knew the word *three*. Madame Peronet had a dinosaur of a computer and painfully slow dial-up internet, so we tried to communicate through terrible online translation services a few times before giving up. There were a handful of other American students in the same program, but the trip was structured in such a way that I rarely saw them. I spent most of my days excruciatingly aware of my loneliness.

The idea of spending springtime in Paris sounds romantic and exhilarating, but I hated it at first. I'd never traveled by myself before, never been so far from home. And there I was, alone in a foreign country, before the days of high-speed internet access, FaceTime, and smartphones. I couldn't afford the cost of international service on my cheap prepaid plan, so I didn't call or text home at all while I was there. I'd picked up enough survival French to get where I needed to go and sort of figure out if my host mom was offering dinner, but that was it. I cried every day for the first two weeks because I was so bitterly lonely and overwhelmed by navigating life in a foreign country.

For the first time in my life, I had nothing to offer. I wasn't able to do or give anything to anyone, couldn't work in France, and there was very little required of me beyond participation in my study-abroad program. I just had to keep showing up.

Somewhere along the way, I realized I had no one to talk to but God. So I started talking. Not with the pressured, anxious prayers

8/27/07

Pastor C gave me a hug before he prayed for me today. "You're doing great," he said, drawing deep sobs from the center of me. All I could do was shake my head — he was smiling, all proud of me. He didn't know that I'd cut myself the last 2 nights, that I'd said, "F— you" to you, Lord, that I'd determined that if something doesn't change, I'm done. He didn't know that, just because I can recognize You're still worth praising doesn't mean that I'm better.

God, help me. When he was praying for me, that I would be able to see + hear the truth, all I could pray was, "Please... please... please..." because I know I need to know the truth. I need to know it, not just hear it + say it. I need to know that there really is a future and a hope that I can look forward to. That You love me. When will I believe this? This is Christianity 101, that You love us. Why should that be so hard? Why should it be that every day is a conscious choice whether or not I will live or die? Deliver me from the cage in my mind that is so terribly persuasive. If I could believe You love me for him to make me better, but about little things: the baguette and bowl of hot chocolate Madame Peronet gave me for breakfast each day, my morning thoughts, my questions as I explored a new city and culture. I spoke with God as I wandered cobblestone streets and bent back alleys, immersed in a world that seemed much older than the one I'd always known.

Something about the cathedrals, with their quiet, cavernous spaces and smooth stone, captivated me. I stood in the cathedral in Chartres, heard the tour guide say the first church on that site had been built by the fourth century, looked up in awe at the building that was now there and had stood since the 1200s. I thought of people living sixteen hundred years before me, in a world that looked so different, trying to love and follow Jesus, just like me.

I lingered over trinkets in the gift shop, absently picking up candles and necklaces. But then a small book with an English title caught my eye: *The Practice of the Presence of God* by Brother Lawrence. "It is God who paints himself in the depths of our soul," the back cover said, promising it would help me feel "His loving presence throughout each simple day."[1] Someone poked his head into the gift shop and said it was time to go. I fished a few euros out of my purse and paid for the book.

Soon after, I was strolling the Left Bank in Paris when I got caught in a downpour. I ducked into Shakespeare and Company, an iconic monastery-turned-bookstore, to escape the rain. As I meandered floor-to-ceiling bookshelves under warm lamplight, I found myself drawn to the mystics and contemplatives throughout Christian history. As I read the words of Brother Lawrence, Jeanne Guyon, Julian of Norwich, Thomas Merton, Henri Nouwen, and others, I learned of ancient Christian prayer practices that were vastly different from anything I'd ever known.

In one of the books, I read the words, "To pray is to descend with the mind into the heart, and there to stand before the face of the Lord, ever-present, all-seeing, within you."[2] These types of prayers seemed so strange, full of stillness and imagery and imagination, but something in them kept calling to me. I wanted God to paint himself within my soul, to find him ever present within me.

So I began to practice this new old kind of prayer. I began sitting alone in my tiny room, windows open, the noise of the city pouring in. I closed my eyes and imagined descending a staircase inside me, making my way from my head to my heart, and meeting a loving, kind Jesus there. When some sort of thought or distraction came up, I pictured it like a rock dropped into a pond, like one of the books had said. Eventually, the ripples from the thought dissipated, and I could gently turn my attention back to Jesus.

My heart, which was so accustomed to racing and rattling in my chest, slowed to a steadier rhythm. I began to breathe more deeply. Prayer stopped feeling so frantic, as though I had to do all the right things to please God. Instead, I began connecting with God in a new way.

There were many days I struggled to pray like this. It wasn't always easy. But over time, it wore away at me, reshaping my soul as water reshapes canyons. Soon, those fevered, pressured prayers—the ones that felt so dependent on me being good enough to get an answer—rarely found their way to my lips. Instead, I chatted quietly with God, told him about my day as well as my pain and heartaches, learned to lament, and learned to listen.

One weekend, I took a trip to Wales, rode a train out to a small town, and found myself in a worship service that felt more like a rave than church. I was used to passionate, expressive worship from my charismatic church back in Oregon, but this seemed rowdy even to me. I perched on a metal folding chair in a crowd of strangers, feeling a little spiritual whiplash after spending a few weeks learning to pray in quiet, peaceful ways. But somewhere between the loud music and ecstatic dancing, I heard somebody share the gospel as though I'd never heard it before. She preached from the verse that says "I have been crucified with Christ. It is no longer I who live, but Christ who lives in me" (Galatians 2:20) and Romans 6:3–10, about being united with his death through baptism. Something about it was different than "Jesus loves you and died for you so you don't have to go to hell."

I had believed that the pain inside me—what I experienced and described as darkness—was actually spiritual darkness that coursed through me like an uncontrolled wildfire, and that God had abandoned me to it. I'd believed that I was too lost, too broken, and too toxic to really be wanted and cared for by a loving God. But as I sat on that hard folding chair, I heard something different: Jesus came to be fully united with us, to take all our brokenness and sin and pain into himself. She talked about all the sin sickness being crucified on the same cross, with the same nails that pierced Jesus. All the things I thought were keeping God away, all the reasons I thought he couldn't possibly love me, were the very things he took onto himself.

And suddenly, I felt it. I experienced the love of God in a way I couldn't deny, and I knew in the deepest part of me that the Jesus who I had committed my life to actually cared about and wanted *me*. I sat there feeling quiet and still, like I could finally relax and let my guard down. It was something like a deep breath, like stretching and stirring after a luxurious afternoon nap. It had happened slowly and then all at once, this realization that my deepest, truest identity is that I am, as Henri Nouwen said, "the Beloved of God."[3]

A week later, I boarded another train for Taizé, a monastery in central France, for a weekend of quiet contemplation. Protestant and Catholic monks live together, where visitors from all over the world are welcome to stay and join in the simple, rhythmic community life. In stark contrast to the wild, loud, charismatic meetings from the week before, worship in Taizé looked like simple songs and chants in many languages interspersed with plenty of silence.

But as I sat in the quiet that first night, surrounded by worshippers and yet hearing nothing but my own breath, I was aware of a simple truth I hadn't believed for the first five years of my faith: I was, and am, deeply loved and fully accepted by God, just as I am. And there was the answer to that prayer my friend had told me to pray so many months before. I had experienced the love of God in a way I couldn't deny.

It took my getting halfway around the world before I could stop trying so hard to perform, to be still long enough to hear the voice of love that had been speaking to me all along.

5/24/08
Taizé

Here, in the place of stillness, we must be honest with you. There's no music, no program, no real excuse to hide behind—it's just You and me. And if I want to seek you out, all I have to do is be still and know—recognize, experience—that You are God and You are in me, bringing Your entire kingdom into my heart. It's simple, so simple. There is no striving not to know You. You're always here inside of my heart, whether circumstances seem ideal to pray or like a big mess. And because of that, I can carry hope around inside of me. Has it always been so simple?

5/25/08
Evening Prayer

I think I just realized this is what this whole European adventure has been about. Not about serving or working but learning to depend on You, to believe that I am loved, and that the plans You have for me are written in the desires of my heart. I know you delight in me.

Depression is different when you don't hate yourself. Angela was right: I really *did* need to know, in the deepest part of me, that God loved me. As my relationship with God healed, I began to see myself with new eyes. I wasn't the toxic, shameful failure I'd always believed I was. The answer to that prayer came nearly ten months after we started praying. But really accepting that love and integrating it into my beliefs about myself was an even longer process. It took years, as I continued to practice stillness and meditation (and eventually went to a lot of therapy), but I began to see the image of God when I looked in the mirror. I began to realize that I am the beloved of God.

I couldn't have foreseen the domino effect of something as simple as learning to be loved by God. What I didn't expect is that when I began to see myself as God saw me, it became much easier to treat myself with kindness. It changed my willingness to practice self-care and set boundaries and helped me realize that God's dreams for me are full of kindness and hope, regardless of whether I'm completely healed or not. More than that, this is when I realized God is with me in the darkness and that he won't leave me, no matter what I do or how angry I get with him.

Understanding my belovedness changed so much for me. I discovered what people mean when they say they find their identities in Christ. There would be years of learning the skills I needed to get well, and there were bumps along the way. But when I eventually slipped back into a deep and terrifying depression, I realized I was worth getting help. So I committed to doing whatever it takes to get better. Over time, that decision led me to finally find a great therapist, get on the medications I needed to get stable, and work through past trauma in therapy. This rich, beautiful, full life I have can, in many ways, be traced back to my relationship with God being healed through prayer and meditation.

Meditation in Scripture

Many Christians argue against meditative practices because they think they're intrinsically new age or heretical. Because other religions also use types of meditation, there's this misconception that meditation and contemplative prayer is inherently bad. I had believed this for a long time too. But if we believe that, we miss out on the beautiful heritage of contemplative prayer that is seen throughout the Bible. Scripture is full of examples of prayer that go far beyond the list of requests that we so often think of. Here are just a few examples of contemplation and meditation in Scripture:

Genesis 24:63—And Isaac went out to meditate in the field toward evening.

Psalm 63:6 (NLT)—I lie awake thinking of you, meditating on you through the night.

Psalm 77:11–12 (NLT)—I recall all you have done, O LORD; I remember your wonderful deeds of long ago. They are constantly in my thoughts. I cannot stop thinking about your mighty works.

Psalm 145:5 (NLT)—I will meditate on your majestic, glorious splendor and your wonderful miracles.

Luke 2:19—But Mary treasured up all these things, pondering them in her heart.

Philippians 4:8 (NLT)—Fix your thoughts on what is true, and honorable, and right, and pure, and lovely, and admirable. Think about things that are excellent and worthy of praise.

The word used in many of these places can be translated to mutter, murmur, muse, or even imagine. It creates a picture of turning something over and over in your mind, or "chewing on it," by reciting it to yourself. This is a prayer of focus—choosing to turn attention back to God and his love and kindness over and over again.

Many of the references to meditation are in Psalms, the book of prayer and worship. David, who struggled with sorrow and despair (if not outright depression, which seems pretty likely), talks often about meditating and returning his attention to God. Over and over, in the midst of discouraging circumstances, contemplating

God's love, goodness, and the good things he's done leads to hope, healing, and a better perspective of ourselves as his beloved.

What Science Says About Prayer

Before I relearned to pray, I thought I was doing everything right to connect with God. But as Dr. Curt Thompson wrote, sometimes we "believe that [we've] been working hard to change, but in fact are quite mistaken. [We] may have been working hard but, unbeknownst to [us], working in ways that reinforce" the patterns that have been keeping us bound.[4] This can absolutely be the case with prayer. My old prayer habits—transactional instead of relational, focused on a God who doesn't *really* love me—were actually plunging me deeper into the darkness.

But our brains have this incredible trait called neuroplasticity; in the simplest terms, it's an ability to change. Scientists talk about neurons and synapses, but laypeople might say we can rewire our brains. While scientists used to believe that the brain couldn't change much after childhood, recent research has demonstrated that even adults can change the structures and connections in their brains. And those changes can significantly impact mental health.[5] This is huge news for those of us who struggle with the darkness. While we may not be able to completely erase old, ingrained pathways, we can develop new thought patterns and practices that grow stronger over time.

And we can actually rewire our perceptions of God to better line up with the truth of who he is. Dr. Andrew Newberg, a neuroscience researcher and author of *How God Changes Your Brain,* discovered that the things we focus on become more real to us as they are written into the connections in our brains.[6] Our minds often can't tell the difference between reality and the perceptions that have been wired into our brains through experiences. That's why when two people read the same Bible passage, one reader interprets it through the lens of a loving, compassionate God while the other interprets it through the lens of a harsh, wrathful God. And our interpretation deeply impacts our mental health.

Dr. Newberg advocates for meditation on the loving, compassionate traits of God for a few reasons. We can change our relationship with and understanding of God by the things we focus on. It turns out that most Americans—72 percent, according to a study by Baylor University—see God as critical, authoritarian, or distant. Those perceptions of God are associated with parts of the brain associated with anger and fear. I know well how severe depression reinforced a perception of God that left me feeling anxious, guilty, and shameful.

Only 23 percent of Americans see God as kind, gentle, and forgiving. What's wild is that perceiving God this way activates a different part of the brain—one linked to empathy, love, and compassion. That part of the brain—known as the anterior cingulate—calms us, reducing feelings of anger, guilt, anxiety, and fear.[7] When we pray and meditate on the truly kind, truly loving character of God, we can strengthen the anterior cingulate. Plus, there's evidence that meditation increases neurotransmitters (chemicals in the brain) that can be deficient in people with mental illnesses, so it's been found to be especially helpful in serious depression.[8]

Researchers are finding that simply focusing or meditating on a loving, gracious God consistently can change our brains and make us actually feel closer to him. As we contemplate the vast love of a God who would leave heaven to be with us, we also begin to see ourselves in a different light: as God's precious, deeply beloved children and friends.

(Re)Learning to Pray

This may sound like a lot to take in, but it's super simple to practice. It literally takes just minutes a day. It can be done in bed on the days when you don't think you can get up, when racing thoughts keep you from falling asleep, on your commute, or even at your desk at work. Those are just some of the places I've practiced it.

Over the years, I have used different methods to practice contemplative prayer. All that matters is that you find one that works for you. One important thing to recognize: your mind will wander.

That's normal and okay—you're not trying to stop thinking other thoughts. There's no reason to beat yourself up over it.

Instead, each time you notice your thoughts wandering, just gently turn your focus back to God. It helps me to picture distracting thoughts like a rock thrown into a still lake. It makes a splash and a ripple, but the ripple soon fades and the water becomes smooth as glass again. Some days, the distracting thoughts will float by occasionally, while others, they'll fill your mind and you'll be turning your attention back over and over. It's absolutely normal.

We call meditation and contemplation a practice because it's something best done over and over, every day. There is no "perfect" prayer, so instead we practice. Take a few minutes—even just five to start. I love to find spare moments throughout my day to close my eyes, breathe deep, and turn my attention to the love of God.

Here Are a Few Options to Try

When you feel alone or rejected, try Brennan Manning's simple prayer practice:[9]

- Sit in a quiet place, with your hands palms up on your lap in a receiving position.
- Either out loud or in your head, repeat, "Abba, I belong to you."
- "Abba" is a biblical term of endearment for a father, like Papa or Daddy. If it's tough to connect with God as a father, you can substitute "Jesus" or "God" or whatever you like for "Abba."

When words fail you, try breath prayer.

- Pick a word or short phrase that represents how you want to connect with God, like "God is love," "Thank you for your grace," or "You are my peace." (My favorite is "You are with me.")

- Close your eyes and sit quietly.
- When you inhale, say the first part of the phrase to yourself.
- When you exhale, say the rest of the phrase.
- Inhale: *You are . . .*
- Exhale: *with me.*
- Repeat this as you breath naturally and calmly, focusing on the love of God and using the phrase to help keep your thoughts from wandering.

When unwanted images or memories haunt you, use your imagination and create a scenario like this:

- Using your imagination is a time-honored way to connect with God. It doesn't mean you're "fooling yourself" or "pretending."
- I like to imagine a specific place that feels safe and peaceful. For me, that's a beautiful garden.
- Picture Jesus meeting you there, spending time with you, and enjoying being close to you.
- I imagine the love in his eyes and the smile on his face, and I sit quietly with him.
- Sometimes I pray a simple phrase, like "I love you, Jesus" or "Thank you for your love."
- As you connect with the feeling of being fully accepted and loved, recognize that this is the truth of who you are.

When the harsh voice of shame is especially loud, allow yourself to feel God's delight.

- This exercise is taken from *Anatomy of the Soul.*[10]
- Zephaniah 3:17 (NIV) says, "The LORD your God is with you, the Mighty Warrior who saves. He will take great delight in you; in his love he will no longer rebuke you, but will rejoice over you with singing."
- Get comfortable and still.

- "Simply imagine, the best that you can, being in God's presence *while he is feeling delighted to be with you.*"[11]
- Then, imagine God so happy to be with you that he starts singing.
- Try to imagine the details—what God would look like, sound like, and say.
- What does that feel like?

When you struggle to focus and need some extra help, use a guided meditation or visualization.

- Search online for "Christian guided meditation" or "Christian contemplative prayer." There are a lot of options on YouTube.
- Download the free Insight Timer app and search for "Christian centering prayer."
- I also love the Abide app—it has a free trial before you need to sign up for a subscription, but it's a great resource for Christ-honoring meditation. I've also heard great things about the Soultime app, though I haven't tried it out myself.

Two other prayer practices have been instrumental to learning how to live well despite severe depression. First is good, old-fashioned lament. When I had nobody but God to talk to in Paris, even before I discovered contemplative prayer, I started talking to him as if he was a friend. When I was angry and hurting, I talked to him about it, but for the first time, I wasn't just begging him to fix it. I was telling him about my pain and inviting him into it. There's something powerful about getting honest, raw, and real before God, just as we would with our dearest loved ones. When I learned to lament, to express the ache of my heart, I leaned into Scriptures like Psalm 13:1 ("How long, O Lord?") and began to see that I could be honest with God about my pain, that he would be right there with me in it.

The other practice that has been essential to me is prayer journaling. Sometimes I'll journal before I sit in silence with God, while other times I'll practice contemplative prayer and then write about things that came up or stuck out to me during that time. When I'm upset, I often go to my journal and pour words on the page, letting them spill out of me without censoring or questioning. That's actually the easiest way for me to lament, to pour out my aches, and to surrender them to God. I have dozens of notebooks, filled with questions, prayers, longings, and doubts. I love looking back at them when I'm discouraged or struggling because I can see ways God has been faithful to me in the past.

Modern, Western, evangelical faith is very solution and answer oriented. We focus on moments and signs and proofs: a single moment of conversion, a miraculous healing, an answer from God that fixes everything. And for many of us, we expect prayer to follow the same pattern. We expect that our requests will be answered.

But God isn't our fixer, cleaning up messes and making life easy for us on our way to the top. He's God. He's mysterious and majestic, loving and beautiful and intimate. He's worthy of love and adoration and trust because of his character, not because of the things he gives us and does for us. When we learn to pray in ways that aren't transactional, when we learn to release our expectations for God to respond in a certain way, the doors open to a healing, life-giving relationship with the Lord.

And so it was that I found a truer experience of God through believers from faith traditions very different from my own. I discovered a God of love, presence, and tender care in the writings of ancient and medieval mystics as well as through modern contemplatives. John of the Cross, Brother Lawrence, Julian of Norwich, Thomas Merton, and Henri Nouwen revealed God in ways I'd never seen. I tried practicing contemplative prayer, leaving behind the endless, desperate begging for healing, and learning to "descend with the mind into the heart."

For me, this happened halfway around the world, cut off from everybody I knew and loved, and unable to do much of anything. But the specifics of my experience aren't what mattered—otherwise we couldn't hope to replicate this type of healing, restorative relationship with God. We must be careful not to elevate specific experiences and special moments into something to be sought after and replicated.

Instead, it is in the place of vulnerable, relational prayer that we are able to connect with a God who is present even in the darkness, even when nothing makes sense.

If you can relate to prayer as a time of desperately begging for something to change in your life, maybe it's time to let that practice go for a while. Instead, I invite you to a new practice—one that isn't just woven throughout Scripture and hasn't just changed my life, but has been scientifically proven to reduce depression and anxiety and literally change your brain. It isn't an instant fix, but it's worth committing to the process to find a God who is ever present inside your heart, ever kind, and ever patient with your pain.

Five

Bad Therapy

I was afraid of therapy. To some extent, this is pretty normal. Many people feel anxious about the idea of going to counseling, if only because it's unknown or it's scary to think about digging up painful thoughts and memories. But my fears went much deeper.

At the time, my church was making some incredible strides toward health and balance. When I first came to faith in that church years before, many people would talk about depression and anxiety as signs of sin or lack of faith. Eventually, as we dismantled some of those unhealthy beliefs, counseling became more widely accepted. Chris and Jenny were the senior pastors now, and I had taken over the youth ministry a few months after returning from Paris. They were a joy to work with; their constant hunger to love and lead well inspired me, and I watched them learn from some hard knocks in ministry. Shifting the emphasis of a church was difficult, but there was a new level of freedom to admit when we weren't okay and didn't have all the answers.

The deep respect I had for my pastors meant that I listened when Chris noticed I was struggling again and suggested that I talk to somebody.

But there were still lingering traces of stigma that made it hard to get help. I still expected God to be my healer—hadn't he answered that prayer in Paris?—and I had internalized a subtle mistrust of science that can be common in evangelical culture. Since high school, I'd often been warned of the dangers of the "wisdom of this world" and ideologies designed to turn Christians away from the Lord. At best, people who held this worldly wisdom wouldn't understand my relationship with Jesus. At worst, I'd been told that if I didn't carefully guard my heart and mind, I'd lose my faith.

It was hard enough to admit I wasn't okay and I needed help or that the support available through my church was insufficient. It wasn't just that I believed it was a lack of faith to look to therapists (let alone doctors) to deal with my head and my heart. It's that I was actually afraid of what they would tell me. I thought they'd think I was crazy. I thought they'd try to undermine my faith or, worse, lock me up if I said something about "hearing from God."

Looking back now, it seems so strange that such fear of science held me back from getting the help I needed. It took a trusted leader encouraging me to seek help and take care of myself before it seemed worth the risk. I started looking into Christian counselors in the area. *Surely if they're Christian counselors, it will be better,* I thought. I didn't know what to look for or how to tell if a counselor or therapist would be a good fit. I would eventually find and work with incredible, Christ-honoring, skilled therapists, but not before some very difficult experiences.

So I found myself sitting in a tiny office across from a woman I'd never met before, trying to tell some cohesive story about why I was there. It was awful. She was so pushy and aggressive. She seemed much less concerned with caring for me as a client than telling me all the actions I needed to take immediately to fix things for other people. I was too scared to ever go back.

At the same time, there was a glimmer of hope: a few comments the counselor had made *were* actually helpful. Despite her aggressive approach, those few words started to normalize my experiences. Even though I knew she wasn't the right fit for me, I was willing to try again.

Trying Again

I'd made the mistake the first time of not asking around or getting recommendations from people I knew, so the second counselor I saw came on a dear friend's recommendation. He hadn't worked with her personally but knew her husband and had heard she was a psychologist. Her website said she was a "licensed clinical Christian counselor" with a "PhD in Christian Psychology" and "board certi-fied," so everything sounded as though it was in order, even though I'd never heard of the college she had attended. I had no idea how misleading those "credentials" were.

I was hopeful that this time would be different. I was a little con-fused when she wanted to spend several sessions working through a temperament test that was supposed to make it easier for her to help me. I dutifully answered questions, listened to explanations, and waited for us to start digging into the issues I struggled with.

As sessions went on, I felt more and more uncomfortable with the fact that my counselor rarely asked any questions. I thought I was supposed to go to counseling to talk, but I couldn't get a word in edgewise. Instead, she talked about herself and the problems in her relationship with her son. I felt like I was floundering.

Over and over, I wrote in my journals that I felt guilty and that I wasn't doing well enough: *God, I feel like I'm failing, like I'm not doing well in my process—why can't I just get it over with? I'm an adult now, a leader at church and at work. I should be so far beyond this.*

After a few months of this, I knew something needed to change. I gathered all my courage as I sat in the parking lot before my next appointment. Still, my heart was in my throat when I told my coun-selor that I didn't feel like I was making progress or getting the help I needed. She didn't miss a beat.

"It's your fault that I can't help you," she said. I felt as though I'd been slapped. "You keep putting up stop signs every time I try to ask anything." She paused as I stared across the desk. "Tell you what, why don't you take the next two weeks and think about whether you want to do this or not."

I never went back. When she said, "I can't help you," I heard, "You're too messed up." As hurtful as the experience was, she was telling the truth. Despite the official-sounding credentials, she wasn't equipped to counsel somebody with a mental health condition.

The Problem with "Biblical Counseling"

At the time, I didn't know that the same underlying fear of science that had kept me from seeking help had birthed a whole stream of so-called counselors who lack any training in psychology, human development, or healthy communication. It's sometimes called nouthetic or biblical counseling, and the key idea behind it is that the Bible holds answers to everything we need in life. On the surface that sounds great, but it breaks down when we begin to consider the implications.

I absolutely love the Bible. I hold it in high esteem and take great joy in connecting with God through Scripture. But I also recognize that it was never intended to be a medical or scientific text. It doesn't tell us how to perform lifesaving open-heart surgery. It doesn't explain how to treat diabetes, cancer, or Alzheimer's disease. It also doesn't tell us how to treat mental illness or trauma.

The second counselor I saw most likely believed the best way she could serve the body of Christ was to pursue an entirely biblically based curriculum. On one occasion, she told me to "ask God what is the lie [I'm] believing and what truth it should be replaced with." She also suggested that when difficult thoughts or memories surfaced, I should "ask God where he was in it." To be fair, it was a nice mental image to think about God being present when I was hurting, and questions like these can be helpful tools when properly applied. But because she wasn't *actually* trained in psychology or mental health counseling, she wasn't able to help me identify the lies I believed or recognize the symptoms of mental illness.

The situation with nouthetic or biblical counseling is complicated by the fact that there is no consistent legal definition of a counselor. In my home state (and most U.S. states), licensing requirements don't apply to "a recognized member of the clergy, provided that the person is acting in the person's ministerial capacity."[1] That means that from a legal standpoint, *anybody* can claim to be a counselor, especially if she's involved in ministry.

At the time, I didn't know that the organization that accredited my second counselor's degree had been shut down for signing off on fake colleges. I didn't know that there are countless Christian schools that offer easy-to-receive degrees that lack academic rigor, trained faculty, or any nationally recognized accreditation. I didn't know that anybody can call himself a biblical counselor or pastoral counselor without any training or oversight whatsoever to protect clients and ensure they receive adequate care.

It's All My Fault

Cultural stigma around mental illness makes it hard to get help. When I sought help and was told it was my fault I wasn't getting better, I was crushed. That message only served to reinforce the lie that I was too broken, too messed up, to ever get better. I still didn't understand that I was dealing with an illness and not a character defect, so that shame loop kept playing. I believed that if these counselors couldn't help me, I must be hopelessly broken.

It would be years before I would try to go to therapy again. In the meantime, I filled my journal with prayers and Bible verses as I fell back on the old belief that I could just "declare healing over myself" and eventually it would stick. Instead of holding Scripture as a weapon against the darkness, I turned it against myself. While journaling Scripture helped remind me of things that are true and good—a God who was present in my pain and remained consistent regardless of my struggles—I was trying to use it to beat my soul into submission and make myself better. I was convinced that I wasn't getting better because of my "inability to let God in." And that's also what I believed about my counseling process: I wasn't doing a good job. I wasn't moving on quickly enough. I wasn't taking the right steps.

Good Gifts and Good Fruit

A multitude of reasons kept me from seeking help for years. First, that mistrust of science translated into a fear of finding answers outside the Bible. But this fear is not biblically founded. Mistrust of science is not rooted in Scripture; neither is the stigma around depending on professionals and other natural means for help. On the contrary, through-out the Bible, we see people seeking wise counsel and support.

But, more than that, by resisting therapy, I was rejecting something good. James 1:17 says that every good gift comes from a good Father. Every single good thing in this world, in our lives, is a gift of grace from a loving God who sends refreshing rain and causes the sun to rise on each of us, regardless of whether we follow him or not (Matthew 5:45). Though our world is broken and sin sick, it's still woven through with immeasurable beauty and wisdom that comes straight from a good God. Theologians call this idea common grace, and we can all experience the benefits of these gifts that are common to humanity.

As an aside, common grace doesn't mean it's equally distributed to all people; we can see that people born into different circumstances around the world experience different access to things God intended to bless mankind (like natural resources, just government, or technological advances). From the beginning of Genesis, God has made it clear that when he gives gifts to people, he also gives the responsibility and freedom to steward those gifts, and sometimes we don't do that in a just and loving way.

Knowledge, insight, and science aren't to be feared; on the contrary, they are all part of that common grace. That includes advances in the field of mental health; we are learning things now that have the potential to alleviate great suffering. Matthew 7:17 tells us that good trees bear good fruit; we can see the good fruit in the lives of people who have received good, professional counseling and learned to live well as a result. With this perspective, it's clear that well-equipped counselors and therapists who help us move toward wholeness are a gift to humanity. We don't have to be suspicious or afraid of psychology because it simply helps us understand how God made us and how we can live the lives he dreams for us.

Why Relationship Matters

Hearing it was my fault I couldn't get better crushed me. It would be a few years before I would be ready to try again. In that time, depressive episodes came and went like tides washing over me, but I was determined to handle them on my own. I couldn't bear the thought of exposing my pain to somebody else who would blame me like that. I moved to a new city and started working with another ministry; eventually, the depression ceased to be a series of manageable tides and rushed in like a flood. I was drowning again, and no matter what I tried, I couldn't claw my way back to the surface. My peers and leaders at my new church begged me to see a counselor; when I was hesitant, a friend helped me set up an appointment.

The third therapist I saw was well equipped, professionally licensed, and kind. She was gentle, warm, and welcoming, and the first time I saw her I could tell she knew her stuff. However, she was also working on staff at a very large church and had multiple obligations. I didn't discover this until I would show up for sessions and she wouldn't. She was often pulled into meetings with the pastoral team, or her assistant sometimes double-booked her calendar. Each time this happened, I was confused and hurt. I carried so much anxiety from prior attempts at working with counselors, and this reinforced my fears. Maybe I wasn't important enough for her to show up for me. Maybe there was something wrong with me. After a couple of experiences like this, I stopped going back. Looking back, I imagine she was overwhelmed and overworked in her role as a staff counselor for a megachurch. But I needed somebody who could be present and consistent. Even though she was a great therapist, her schedule during that season meant she wasn't the right fit for *me*.

Those hurtful experiences became a breeding ground for lies I began to believe about myself, about God, and about what it meant to be a follower of Christ. In retrospect, I can see what I was unable to recognize then: those devastating experiences were not a reflection of me. They were a reflection of either an ill-equipped therapist or a simple mismatch. That issue—a mismatch—is one that's well researched and understood in the mental health community. In fact, research has found that a good match between the client and therapist is the biggest predictor of successful treatment.

My current counselor (whom I love and will talk more about in the chapter on working with a therapist) often says that 90 percent of the success of therapy lies in the relationship between the client and therapist. Studies have found that "factors such as empathy, warmth, and the therapeutic relationship" are more linked to positive outcomes in therapy than any special techniques or approaches."[2] Mental health professionals agree; another study found the majority of clinicians believe the "therapeutic alliance" is the most important factor in the success of therapy.[3] The bottom line is that while there are many styles, techniques, and modalities, what matters most is a good working relationship with your therapist.

How to Find a Great Therapist

For many, a huge barrier to assembling a professional support team is not knowing what to look for. Maybe, like me, you've had some bad experiences with counselors who weren't the right fit or weren't well equipped to help you. I know how discouraging and painful that can be. But I also want to give you hope: there are incredible professionals with God-given gifts in counseling who can help you walk the path toward wholeness. For now, if you aren't working with a skilled therapist you feel safe with, here are some tips on how to find a good one.

Consider Your Specific Needs and Circumstances

Not every counselor is trained for the specific challenges you experience. I've discovered that working with a trauma-informed therapist is much more effective for me than a general mental health counselor. You can find specialists in many areas, including the following:

- major depression
- suicide
- grief and loss
- addiction
- child or adolescent therapy

- trauma
- postpartum depression
- abuse (including childhood abuse or sexual abuse)
- marriage and family issues
- sexual issues
- cultural competence

You may also have some specific needs or preferences, such as working with a counselor of the same gender or making sure he's culturally competent (that means he's trained and aware of cultural differences that could impact therapy and is able to adapt in a way that serves you).

Consider Your Budget

Many people don't pursue therapy because they believe they can't afford it. I understand this, and there have been many times I wasn't sure I could justify the cost out of pocket. But working with a compassionate, well-equipped therapist can be life altering in the best way; it's absolutely worth the cost. I've also discovered tons of options available to help you afford good help.

- If you have insurance, ask your insurance company for its full list of mental health providers and details on covered services (for example, how many appointments).
- Check with your HR department to see if your employer offers an employee assistance program (also called EAP) and see what services are included.
- Search "sliding scale counseling in (your city)." For years, I saw therapists on a sliding scale, which means the fee was adjusted to fit my income.
- If you live near a university with a graduate program in counseling, psychology, or social work, reach out to see what options it has. In my city, there is a program where you can work with newly licensed therapists for as little as $5 per session, based on your income.

- Look into online or virtual therapy. While I still see my local counselor, some of my friends rave about online services such as BetterHelp or Talkspace, which provide a subscription-based therapy service. A month of virtual therapy can cost less than a single in-person session.

Ask Around

More and more people are going to counseling these days. I'm thrilled to see more comments about it on social media and hear people mention it in casual conversation. If you've heard somebody mention a good counselor, ask her for a recommendation. Here are some other ways you can use your network to find a good counselor:

- Ask your doctor.
- If you don't want to see the same person as a friend or family member (whether because you want someone who specializes in your challenges or just somebody separate from your social circle), that's okay. Get the name of the provider, then reach out and see if that person will recommend other local therapists.
- Do you know anybody in the mental health field? Ask for a referral (you shouldn't see a counselor you know socially).

Search Online

Once you've gone through the previous steps, you might still need a few names. PsychologyToday.com has an incredible detailed therapist finder that lets you filter by specialty, insurance accepted, gender, language, and more.

Reach Out and Ask Questions

Once you've got the list in hand, it's time to reach out. I know this is hard and feels scary; there have been times I've waited days or

weeks before sending an email or making a call. Here are questions
to consider asking the providers:

- Do they offer consultations? (Some do for free, others
  don't. It's helpful, but not necessary, in my experience.)
- How long have they been practicing?
- What is their style or approach like? If they tell you they
  use a specific technique but you're not sure what it is, don't
  be afraid to ask for clarification.
- Do they offer telehealth or virtual therapy?
- Are they culturally competent? (This can be especially important for members of historically underrepresented communities, as therapists from different backgrounds may
  not be aware of cultural differences and privileges that can
  damage the therapeutic relationship and hinder the client's
  progress.)
- What do they expect from clients? What can clients expect
  from them?
- What do boundaries look like in working with them?
- What types of clients do they work best with?
- When do they refer clients to other professionals?
- Do they or have they gone to therapy? (You can also ask if
  they are seeking supervision from another therapist and, if
  not, under what circumstances they would. Supervision is
  simply consulting with an experienced, wise therapist who
  acts as a confidential consultant to help your therapist provide great care, deal with blind spots she may have, and
  take care of herself).
- Where did they get their degrees? (If you've never heard of
  the school, either look it up or ask probing questions about
  where it is, what type of school, and whether it's accredited
  through an association like CACREP, which is the top cre-
  dentialing association for counseling graduate programs.)
- Are they licensed? (Verify this with your state's licensing
  board. Search "verify therapist license in [your state].")

- If you have a diagnosis (bipolar disorder, borderline personality disorder, depression, obsessive-compulsive disorder, and so on), what is their experience working with clients with that diagnosis?

Commit to Showing Up

When I see a new therapist, it's tough to tell if it's going to work out right at the beginning, so I don't commit to working with someone long term right away. Assuming there are no major red flags (see below), I commit to showing up for three sessions. That usually gives me enough time to get past the jitters of working with a new person and to see how we mesh. I can then make an informed decision to carry on or move on. The good news is that after implementing the tips outlined above, I've had great success finding therapists I connect well with. Still, setting a low initial commitment makes the process seem a lot less scary.

Notice Red Flags

Here are some of the things to watch out for as you're building a relationship with a new therapist. Some of them are big issues and can be reasons to stop working with that therapist immediately (lack of professional boundaries, breaking confidentiality, inappropriate physical contact, not being present and respectful).

Others aren't as serious and can sometimes be resolved with a conversation. For example, after working with my current counselor for a while, I realized that I needed more time to think and finish sharing before she responded. I shared this with her, and she thanked me for sharing and adjusted her style. The key is that when I brought up a concern, she was respectful, professional, and worked with me on it. If something bothers you but doesn't seem like a major red flag, try a conversation. But if it is unethical or makes you feel unsafe in any way, it's okay to fire your therapist and find a new one.

Here are some red flags:

- Not being present in sessions (eating, texting, not paying attention).
- Talking too much.
- Lacking personal boundaries or not maintaining a professional relationship. (For example, the counselor shouldn't touch or hug you at all without permission, and they should rarely offer or ask.)
- Sharing information about other clients by name (not vague, unidentifiable information told in a helpful context).
- Not going to therapy themselves. (This helps them work through difficult issues that arise in therapy as well as grow through their own blind spots. If they aren't going or haven't gone to therapy quite a bit, they aren't going to be healthy enough to help you get healthier.)
- Having no experience or training with issues specific to you.
- Minimizing your feelings or telling you how you "should" feel.
- Not asking questions; too quick to tell you what to do.
- Showing disrespect for your experiences or thoughts if they are different from theirs.
- Not offering collaboration and room for discussion if you bring up a concern (as I did with my second therapist).
- A therapist should never, under any circumstances, hit on you or pursue any type of personal relationship (sexual, romantic, platonic, or otherwise) outside the professional therapeutic relationship.
- You just don't feel comfortable *enough*. Talking about this stuff is uncomfortable for most people. Especially at first, you'll probably feel shy about opening up completely. But you should feel safe *enough* to keep coming back. If you don't want to return, ask yourself if it's simply the initial discomfort of opening up or if there's something about the way the counselor interacts with you that makes you feel unsafe.

If it takes a while to find the right fit, you might start to feel discouraged. That's totally normal, and there's nothing wrong with you if you don't get a good match after a few tries. It's okay if you need to take a short break before trying again (though I don't recommend waiting years, as I did). If it feels overwhelming, maybe commit to spending five minutes a day researching until you feel able to spend a little more time. And don't be afraid to ask a friend or loved one for help. You could ask her to check on your progress if accountability motivates you, or even ask her to help you find some options and make an appointment if you need that help.

My early experiences with counseling felt devastating at the time because I believed they meant I was too broken to get better. If you've experienced heartache as you've sought help, I'm so sorry. Please don't believe the lies that there isn't good, compassionate help available for you. It may take a little work and you might have to see a few before you find a good one, but there is a mental health professional out there who can help you learn to live well despite the darkness. Don't give up until you find the right fit.

Part Two

SURVIVING

Six

Permission to Be Broken

"Honey, you struggle with depression, don't you?"

My heart fell right through the floor as if it had accidentally wandered into the Tower of Terror. Those words from a mentor, so simple and so compassionate, still managed to cut deep, tearing apart my carefully constructed performance.

The first thing I felt was that familiar shame wrapping around me. Nausea rose in my chest as my thoughts started spinning. Once again, I'd proved unable to fix myself, unable to keep the ache pressed down enough to succeed in ministry. Eight months prior, I'd left the small church where I was a youth pastor and moved across the country to be part of a thriving, internationally recognized ministry. The transition was exciting but difficult; I desperately missed the church I'd loved and served in for years, and the pace of life in a megachurch was grueling. For a while, I thought I'd cracked the code and was past the pain I'd always carried, but the mounting stress had freed me from that illusion. But I couldn't let my guard down. I'd fought so long to keep it together on my own that I counted it failure to be seen as anything but a perfect servant-hearted leader, whether as a small-town youth pastor or as part of a massive ministry team.

But then she continued.

"I know, because I do too. I can tell you live under the cloud, though you fight it valiantly. You haven't just rolled over and died, but it's still there." She went on, telling me I needed to learn to take care of myself, that I would need to prioritize it if I wanted to last in ministry. But my heart was slowly turning over, crawling back up from the pit of my stomach as I realized what she was saying.

I felt hot tears on my face and they tasted like freedom. I still wanted to sink under the table, but something in me sighed with relief. This darkness was depression, named and open and no longer denied. I wasn't used to the vulnerability of brokenness. I was used to pulling in and standing up straight and taking more weight. I had grown accustomed to pushing back, resisting anything that looked like weakness, because that's what I thought would make me better.

But that day, she identified the brokenness I hadn't made peace with. She gave me permission to stop thinking I was failing because I couldn't try my way into restoration.

She told me it was okay to need help. Until this moment, I had believed that I was on my own, that the ability of my brain to create joy was somehow in my control and if I could just pray harder or spend more time in Scripture, it would all be okay.

Sure, I had tried to go to therapy a few times, but that hadn't gone well. And it certainly hadn't lasted long enough for me to come to terms with a diagnosis of depression or accept that it wasn't about my failure. So I'd been left trying to use the old coping skills that had never quite been enough. The more I tried to beat back the darkness with white-knuckle faith, the more it feasted on shame and disappointment. It was a vicious cycle, and I was stuck as long as I refused to accept that I had depression.

When I was a youth pastor at my first church, I didn't have much time for myself. There were just too many commitments to keep, too many people to care for. Starting off in a small ministry meant there wasn't room in the budget for staff salaries, so I worked another full-time job to support myself. I'd spend my lunch breaks and evenings preparing sermons and worship sets for youth-group services. I'd squeeze in coffee dates and small-group sessions, calls with parents and countless meetings. And even though I'd struggled for years, I couldn't admit to myself that I had depression. I'd never talked with a doctor. I still hadn't found a decent counselor. And there were a lot of holdovers from the unhealthy theology of my teen years.

Most of all, I was afraid of being truly honest with myself about the heaviness that lived inside me. In some Christian circles, the verse that says "death and life are in the power of the tongue" (Proverbs 18:21) can be taken too literally. For me, this meant not just hearing that words have power but that anything negative we said about ourselves was essentially a curse. A small part of me still believed that if I said I was sad, let alone depressed or suicidal, I would make it true with my words.

So when those old fears followed me to my new church, I did what I knew to do: I ran as hard as I could, desperately trying to outpace the creeping fog that always caught up. I focused on taking care of those around me, saying yes, and always showing up. There was more to do than I could ever possibly cross off my list: late-night ministry meetings, early mornings setting up for events, eight services each week, and countless people who needed answers, prayer, or comfort.

I loved ministry. When the clouds weren't so heavy, I felt like myself when I poured into the lives of others. I felt like I knew what I was made for in those moments. I just pushed aside the weariness, the emptiness, the sense of there not being quite enough of me to spread around. And I still clung to the lie that if I just tried hard enough, served others well enough, loved Jesus with my life enough, I would be okay. And God would be happy with me.

But denying our circumstances doesn't change them any more than closing our eyes makes the sky disappear. And my circumstances include chronic depression that sometimes goes into remission and sometimes comes roaring back.

Inevitable as the change of seasons, the darkness crept back in. I was too busy to notice the early stages, the gray fog that slowly thickened over my life. *I'm just tired. I need to choose joy,* I'd think, when I finally recognized the way the color had drained from my life. Although "tired" didn't begin to describe the bone-deep weariness and there was no joy to be found, I forced myself to keep going.

When my insides shook and I couldn't catch my breath, I kept going.

When panic attacks set my body on fire and I thought I might die inside the bone-crushing terror, I kept going.

When the abyss in my chest grew so deep I thought I'd fall into it, collapsing on myself, I kept going.

And when ugly thoughts of self-harm and suicide started popping up like a wretched game of whack-a-mole, I kept going.

I've learned that denial is a time thief. It robs us of opportunities to move toward wholeness when we're busily pushing away the reality of our circumstances. I lost years, busily rejecting the reality that I woke up to every day, when embracing depression and accepting that it's an illness would have made a world of difference for me.

Stigma makes this sort of denial a popular pastime in our culture, especially in the church. When we believe good Christians—or pastors, or leaders, or whoever—don't struggle with mental health issues, it's really difficult to open up, admit that we're depressed, and come to a place of acceptance. It can be even tougher for those in leadership positions to share our struggles because we fear being declared unfit for ministry.

The heartbreaking reality is this: as suicide rates continue to grow, nobody is immune. In the church, that means we are losing more and more of those in ministry. The news might stop our breath and make us wonder how somebody who seemed to love and serve people so well could take his own life. Often, you'd never know he was struggling.

That was my story until my wise friend helped me see something crucial about depression: it's an illness, just like any other disease. It's got a serious physical component, including all sorts of physiological causes. I couldn't make it go away through avoidance or wishful thinking any more than I could with any other chronic illness.

All that time, I'd thought acceptance meant giving up without a fight. But it actually meant freedom because I couldn't treat something I ignored, resisted, and fought. It meant taking a crucial step on the long journey to a rich, beautiful life.

Over time, I learned to pay attention to my symptoms because, just as jitters and brain fog can alert a diabetic to low blood sugar, they can be messengers to help me get what I need.

In the years since coming to terms with my depression, medication, lifestyle changes, and lots of prayer have made a world of difference for me. Today, my illness holds a mere shadow of the power it did five or ten years ago. But a great deal of that transformation came about because I accepted the reality that depression and anxiety are part of my life. I will likely live with my diagnoses until the day I go home to Jesus.

That might be your experience too. If it is, you're not alone.

Even if you don't deal with a physical or mental illness, we will *all* live with difficult, imperfect circumstances for the rest of our lives. Some of us carry grief from lost loved ones or broken relationships for years. Others walk with a God who is able to heal and restore but, for whatever reason, doesn't.

And that is a hard thing to accept when everything within us, in all creation, longs for the restoration of these broken things. But as long as we deny and refuse our struggles, we can't address them. As long as we try to resist the pain, it will only intensify. Instead, we need to learn to accept our circumstances without allowing them to drown or control us.

There's this theory in childbirth called the "Fear-Tension-Pain cycle."[1] The idea is that when women experience fear in childbirth, it creates physical tension. That tension is what causes the majority of pain in childbirth. Those tight muscles wind up fighting what the body already knows to do. Most of the pain comes from resisting what's happening in our bodies.

Instead, experts argue that if women are educated on what to expect during labor and learn ways to relax and "lean in" to the contractions, the pain is dramatically lessened. Laboring women will still experience pressure and intense sensations, but they'll perceive less pain. Strange as it sounds, there have even been documented cases of *pain-free birth*—but that happens only when the new mother is able to accept the pressure and challenges of labor without fear and resistance.

Mental and emotional pain is like that too. Admitting our

brokenness—even to ourselves—can be scary. So we can tense up, pushing against the reality of depression, anxiety, grief, or whatever we don't want to face. We run faster, try harder, or we think things like, *Why is this happening to me? I hate this. I can't stand this.* And the pain gets worse.

That's why it's so important for us to give each other the permission to be broken we so desperately need. When those around us aren't afraid to accept our struggles, it makes it easier for us to accept ourselves. When we can lean in to the pressure and ride the waves, we learn to live well, even in the toughest seasons.

Evidence of accepting difficult circumstances is strung throughout Scripture. Job sat in the ashes of his life and grieved without expressing resistance or denial. David refused to fight back against Saul, even though Saul was trying to kill him (1 Samuel 24:10).

But the best biblical example of someone accepting difficult circumstances is Jesus in the Garden of Gethsemane. He knew what was coming: the betrayal by dear friends, the horrific torture, and the anguish of taking every act of evil into himself. Scripture is breathtakingly clear on this fact: he didn't want to go through with it.

In fact, Jesus prayed this in the garden in Luke 22:42: "Father, if you are willing, please take this cup of suffering away from me. Yet I want your will to be done, not mine" (NLT). And though he asked for a way out several times, he accepted that he was about to walk through the worst pain he would ever experience.

Then, in Matthew 26, when the soldiers came to take Jesus away, Peter pulled out a sword to defend him. He managed to cut off somebody's ear before Jesus could tell him to put the sword away. "Don't you realize that I could ask my Father for thousands of angels to protect us, and he would send them instantly?" (verse 53, NLT).

Jesus was telling Peter that as awful as the situation was, it had to be faced and accepted. In this situation, fighting back and resisting wasn't going to work. It wasn't the right thing to do. So Jesus walked through that terrible night of betrayal and beatings without denial or resistance—simply depending on the grace of his Father to carry him through.

We see acceptance as a theme in Paul's life too. He told us about his "thorn in the flesh," something that tormented him but kept him humble. Here's what Paul had to say in 2 Corinthians 12:8–10 (NLT):

> Three different times I begged the Lord to take it away. Each time he said, "My grace is all you need. My power works best in weakness." So now I am glad to boast about my weaknesses, so that the power of Christ can work through me. That's why I take pleasure in my weaknesses, and in the insults, hardships, persecutions, and troubles that I suffer for Christ. For when I am weak, then I am strong.

Whatever this struggle was, God asked Paul to accept it. But the reason behind it is beautiful: God wanted to show his grace and strength to and through Paul's pain and weakness.

I can relate to this. I've prayed many times for God to heal me of my depression, of physical pain, of anxiety. But while I believe God is still able to heal, he hasn't chosen to do it for me. That's why I said earlier that I will probably live with this until I go to be with Jesus.

These days, I'm pretty much okay with that. *Really.*

Don't get me wrong; if Jesus showed up at my door, offering miraculous healing, I'd take him up on it in a heartbeat. Who wouldn't? I would be thrilled to never miss another social event because of a panic attack, never have another thought about hurting myself, never feel the ache that makes it so hard to breathe sometimes.

But instead of offering quick healing that would have been an amazing story, he chose to walk the long road with me. And this is the road that has revealed the unfathomable kindness of Immanuel, God with Us.

His strength—and love, and peace, and immense gentleness toward us—is made complete in our greatest weakness.

This is what Paul meant when he said, "I can do all things through him who strengthens me" (Philippians 4:13). He wasn't talking about winning games or achieving goals. Paul was talking about finding contentment in the midst of really hard situations: he endured shipwrecks, beatings, imprisonment, and starvation.

And he was able to accept his circumstances and see God do amazing things in the midst of them.

> God, grant me the serenity to accept the things I
>   cannot change,
> the courage to change the things I can,
> and wisdom to know the difference.

The Serenity Prayer, originally written in a slightly different form by American theologian Reinhold Niebuhr, has become famous in part because it's become central to Alcoholics Anonymous's recovery process. But it's much more than a few encouraging words. Studies have shown the power of accepting not only our circumstances and life events, but also our emotions. *People who regularly accept their emotions in a nonjudgmental way are more psychologically healthy than those who habitually judge and resist their thoughts and feelings.*[2] The beauty of the Serenity Prayer is that it clarifies a simple issue: some (many) things are outside our control, and those are the things we accept. But it also reminds us that we *can* control how we respond to circumstances.

Acceptance isn't usually a line-in-the-sand moment. Instead, it's a process that develops over time as we move from denial to agency.[3] (Agency is the sense of being in charge of our lives, knowing we can make choices and impact our circumstances.[4]) In other words, accepting our struggles and circumstances—whether it's a mental health diagnosis, a season of grief, or a temporary setback—isn't usually instant and complete. But acceptance actually empowers us to grow, heal, and change.

There's a reason acceptance doesn't come naturally. Our brains and bodies are designed to sound alarms by creating discomfort when something's not right through a pattern of reactions, sensations, and behavior called aversion. It's a brilliantly effective mechanism that pushes us to solve problems and keep ourselves safe. This intense sense of dislike, disgust, or even hate makes us avoid spoiled food, protect ourselves from injury, and try to alleviate pain.

Things get more complicated when we feel aversion to something going on inside us, like depression. Those intense feelings of disgust and hatred might keep us safe from threats on the outside, but we can't fight off or run away from what's going on inside. Still, that's what our bodies do, tensing and bracing as though resistance can save us from our negative thoughts and feelings.[5]

The authors of *The Mindful Way Through Depression* call the aim to get rid of these feelings a "compelling yet futile task." When we can't wrestle depression to the ground as though it were a physical opponent, we're driven to focus on it even more. We find ourselves locked in a battle, convinced the pain we feel is an enemy to be defeated and destroyed. In the process, we lose sight of the choices and options that actually could help us feel better.[6]

It's bizarre that the very thing that feels most natural—resisting and denying that mental illness is part of our existence—actually robs us of our ability to seek wholeness and make the choices we need to get better. Denying depression is like trying to play tug-of-war with a monster. But acceptance is like putting down the rope, allowing the monster to sit there, and taking a good look at it. When we're not fighting so hard, we realize it's not as scary or powerful as we thought.[7] It's still a serious force to be reckoned with, but it doesn't need to control our lives. We can learn to live well with it when we accept its presence.

You might feel unsure about this because acceptance can sometimes seem like loss of hope. If you accept that mental illness is part of life, that it might never go away, then what? Do the years stretch out before us, bleak and unending, without beauty or joy to look forward to?

Thankfully, no. Not at all. Which is good news because who would want that sort of life? No, my friend, acceptance is a key that unlocks incredible potential. Instead of using all that energy on denial and resisting reality, we can redirect it to more productive, life-giving pursuits. We can seek treatment, practice healthy self-care, extend compassion to ourselves, learn to see God in the darkness, and discover beauty in the tiny everyday moments that make up our lives.

Acceptance might not come from a wise friend or mentor for you. It might be something you have to choose daily, over and over. But if you need that permission to be broken, to accept the struggle and the dark, take it from me. You're not a bad person if you're anxious and ache and deal with depression. You're not failing as a Christian, displeasing God, or irreparably broken. It's time to put down that tug-of-war rope. Don't let denial rob you of any more time to move toward wholeness.

Seven

Relapse, Reputation, and Risk

The relapse was as much a surprise to me as it was to those around me. I thought I was better. I was starting to come to terms with the fact that I deal with depression but hadn't figured out that this was a chronic thing, with all the ups and downs that come with it.

I prided myself on my reputation as someone who was wise, emotionally mature, grounded, and strong in my faith. I loved it when people asked for my insight on Scripture and their relationships with God and other people. There's part of my heart that longs to mentor and encourage others, and pouring into youth and young adults fed that part of me.

Maybe it also fed some pride. Or maybe it was just wishful thinking on my part, assuming the ache was behind me.

Then came the relapse.

It seemed so unexpected at the time because I'd thought everything was going so well. But the truth is that I had so many layers of unresolved hurt, decades of pain and lies that I'd come to believe about myself, about God, and about others. Even though I had been given permission to be broken and to do what I needed to take care of myself, I slipped into my old habit of trying to outwork and outrun the darkness. The weight of unrealistic expectations and impossible standards I held for myself started to be a little much to bear.

I loved ministry, but I also looked to it to validate my "enoughness." Underneath my servant-hearted exterior was a fear I would never belong and a desire to work hard enough to earn my keep. I required perfection in my work, that it would far exceed the expectations of those around me, and that it would somehow prove I was really okay. I secretly believed that at my core, I was lazy and incompetent, so I regularly worked at the church until the security guard came to shut things down at ten or eleven at night, even though nobody asked that of me. I lacked balance and boundaries because I found my worth in my ministry work.

At some point, I felt God gently impressing verses upon my heart like Galatians 3:3, where Paul asked, "Are you so foolish? Having begun by the Spirit, are you now being perfected by the flesh?" Part of me understood that this was a call to relax a little, to stop thinking I had to be perfect by my own effort (what Paul called the flesh). I understood, on some level, the call of grace to stop striving so hard, but I constantly beat myself up for not having enough quiet times, not doing enough to change the world, not being a good enough Christian or leader or person. That battle filled the pages of my journal as I fought the idea that it was okay to let my guard down.

I knew I was imperfect. Maybe it was okay to let my guard down and acknowledge my brokenness to my leaders, to people I looked up to. But not to those I served. Not to those who would be rattled to know that somebody *they* look up to struggles.

Even after I experienced the power of vulnerability and permission to be broken, I hesitated to share my battle with mental illness. I still believed that even if I could privately acknowledge my pain and start implementing some minor self-care strategies, it was a leader's responsibility to appear strong and trustworthy. So I just tried to keep up the act.

I don't know why it never occurred to me that others would respond to my revelations of brokenness the way I did when I saw respected leaders share their struggles. When my friend and mentor named depression in me and followed it up with "I know, because I deal with it too," I didn't look down on her. My faith wasn't rattled. Instead, I felt relieved to know somebody else who deeply loved Jesus and tried her best to serve others sometimes felt like I did.

And I'm afraid of the Pit, of descending into something that so blinds me that I refuse your help. I'm afraid I'll start hurting myself again. I'm afraid to feel it all because its more overwhelming + crushing than I can say. And the nightmares. And the fear.

And of being incapacitated by the darkness. So what if my "default" is taking care of people? How wrong can that actually be? I can't afford to become such a mess that I need to step away from ministry again. People depend on me and there are students to disciple + I'm already not doing the best job there.

I want to be able to take care of others, but I really don't want to be taken care of, to be perfectly frank. I <u>don't</u> want to be a burden. I <u>don't</u> want to be selfish + make things about me.

Summer turned to autumn, and the pace of ministry picked up. We started preparing for a flurry of events—the camp our megachurch put on during fall break and back-to-back retreats for youth pastors from around the country. Pressure mounted. The familiar ache returned to my chest. Small decisions seemed overwhelming, and I could barely find the energy to continue going through the motions. I remember sitting on my closet floor for twenty minutes one morning, trying to will myself to move my leaden limbs and put my shoes on.

I couldn't figure out how to keep moving with the heavy fatigue or the hollow numbness inside my rib cage. One of the curses of depression is not knowing whether it's worse to feel dead or be in pain. Depression burns and aches, yes, but it also empties you out. There's this weird, paradoxical disconnect that can make you feel like a disembodied ghost and an abandoned shell where a soul once lived, all at the same time. Something about the experience of this numbness is disorienting, disturbing. As I alternated between that deadened state and all the pain and anger, I couldn't figure out a way to cope. I kept thinking of the way I used to deal with it, the ways I would take those feelings and write them in my skin. I wish I could tell you I resisted by leaning on healthy coping skills I'd learned over the years, by reminding myself of my belovedness and that it was okay to be broken, but I didn't. As the fog closed in around me, I white-knuckled, hanging on by sheer willpower. One night, I rifled through drawers in search of a blade; I held it in my hand for a long moment. I knew if I started cutting, it wouldn't be just once. My heart rattled my ribs like the bars of a prison cell as I tucked the razor away. I sat on the floor of my shower shaking violently, head in my hands. I'd made it through.

But it didn't last. It couldn't last, not when I was depending on strength that seemed to drain out of me more each day. Soon, I was self-harming again.

I don't know if I would have asked for help if Alexis hadn't found me staring vacantly in the kitchen. She lived in the apartment above mine and we often left our doors unlocked. She walked in just moments after I'd finished cutting, and though I had already hidden the wounds, she could see immediately something was wrong. The smile on her face faded quickly.

"Sarah?" She caught my eyes before I looked away. "What's going on?"

A hot wave of nausea hit me. I was supposed to have my act together. *Now I can't pretend.* I was shaking as I prepared myself for the anger and judgment I knew were coming, once I realized I couldn't lie to her.

But the judgment never came. Alexis pulled me into the tiny laundry closet, securing a little privacy from my roommates who could walk in at any moment. I leaned against the wall, then slid to the floor between the washer and dryer. I don't remember what I said or how I told her, but afterward, I remember Alexis saying those same words I'd heard years before: "I'm not disappointed in you." Then she pulled me close and said, "It's okay. We'll figure it out. We'll figure it out," over and over, rubbing my back and stroking my hair.

I'm sure she was shocked to find out I was cutting. I'm sure she didn't have a clue what to do in the moment.

But she did exactly the right thing. She loved me well.

Alexis's gentle response gave me courage. I started admitting to those closest to me (one at a time) that I had relapsed with self-harm, and I was surprised that almost every time, it was well received. There was no shaming, no disappointment (though some sadness and surprise). No anger, no "you should know better" comments.

Around this time, one of my youth-group students was struggling with her mental health. She'd told me her story, talked about the bullying, abuse, and trauma. Like me, she was trying to cope with it through self-harm. I'd told her that I had dealt with depression in the past, that I knew what it was like to go to bed wishing I would never wake up. But not that it was a current battle for me.

One week, she didn't show up to youth group, so I texted her to check in. Her mom responded from her phone, "She tried to kill herself. She's in the hospital." I felt sick, knowing how desperate she must have felt.

A few days later, I was running errands for my job when I got a phone call from an unfamiliar number. When I answered, I was surprised to hear the student's voice on the other end. She sounded tired. I couldn't believe she was using her daily phone time to call me.

I remember standing in Hobby Lobby, quietly confessing that I could relate to her ache more than she could know. I had told her about prior episodes of depression and self-harm. But it was in that paint aisle that I told her I still wrestled with the darkness, that I understood her bad days and thoughts about hurting herself. I flushed hot with embarrassment, thinking somebody else might hear me, but I kept talking. I told her about the day it took me twenty minutes to put on my shoes because it seemed too difficult, the way thoughts of hurting myself pushed unbidden into my mind countless times each day.

I don't know why I was so vulnerable in the moment. I guess I just didn't want her to feel alone. I didn't tell her that I'd relapsed with self-harm or that I was also having suicidal thoughts at the time. But for the first time, I talked about the hard things I dealt with *in the present tense,* not as things I'd "overcome" in the past.

Months later, when she was baptized, she talked about a few people who had made a big impact. She mentioned my name as one of the reasons she was still alive. I was shocked; I had no idea how much sharing my story and letting someone know she's not alone could help.

In the weeks and months after that conversation in the paint aisle of Hobby Lobby, I started opening up more and more. At first, I told myself that my vulnerability might help others, the way it had helped the student. But what started from a desire to be a better leader helped me more than I could have expected. When I talked about my pain, even when I was trying to set an example of vulnerability for others, I was met with grace and encouragement.

At one point, I found myself in a room full of strong, talented, independent young women. We had gone to church and done ministry together for a couple of years by then. I was several years older than they were, and I clung to the notion that I needed to set an example of a wise and mature leader. But something in me knew I needed to let my guard down with them.

I remember being composed and calm when I shared that I was struggling with severe depression, self-harm, and suicidal thoughts. But I burst into tears when I shared my real fear: *Please don't use this against me. Please don't judge me and look down on me.*

I can still see the shock on some of their faces. Then my friend Blake spoke up, talking about her own depression, the sadness that never left. And then another started crying. She told us how she had been planning to end her life because she couldn't handle the pain anymore. I was shocked. I had no idea they were wrestling with the darkness too. Suddenly, I didn't feel so alone.

Soon, there wasn't a dry eye in the room as more of these women shared about the pressure and pain they dealt with. And then the three of us were surrounded as the others placed comforting hands on our backs, embraced us, prayed over us.

———

We always feel alone in the darkness. It's one of the lies of mental illness that sneaks in with all the shame: *Nobody else knows what this is like. I am all alone.* I've believed that lie more often than I can count. I've been surprised to hear it on the lips of friends, of readers, of strangers who also wrestle with their pain.

But Scripture tells us that we don't experience any temptation or trial that isn't common to all of us and that there's nothing new under the sun (1 Corinthians 10:13; Ecclesiastes 1:9). It can be tough to believe, but I find it incredibly reassuring. Specific circumstances may be different, but pain is universal to the human experience. And mental illness is shockingly common; about one out of every five adults in the United States experiences mental illness (that was about 47.6 million people in 2018).[1]

I know it can feel terrifying to speak up. It's always easier when somebody else goes first. Lord knows I still feel more comfortable talking about my own darkness if somebody else has already mentioned his. But we are called, as Christians, to bear one another's burdens (Galatians 6:2). How can we do that if nobody will speak up to share what those burdens are? And that reality goes both ways. I can't share the load of others if they're afraid to speak up, and nobody will come and take some of the weight for me if I keep my mouth shut.

There's a difference between sharing your struggles because you are looking for support and sharing them in order to help others. Because it makes you much more vulnerable to reach out when you're in a crisis and needing help, you need to have a good idea that the person you're opening up to is a safe person. The good news is that people show us who they are through countless tiny everyday clues. Some of them are obvious, while others are a bit more subtle. According to the essential book on the topic, *Safe People*, here are some ways to tell:[2]

- *How do they respond to pain in others?* What did they say when a coworker lost a loved one? How do they handle it when somebody talks about problems in their marriage or a job loss? I'm looking for empathy here. If somebody is quick to make a joke, try to fix it, or explain a problem away, I won't open up when I need support.

- *Have they earned trust in other ways?* Healthy friendships and relationships involve building trust over time, and safe people recognize that. They don't demand trust right away. I don't share my deepest struggles or dark thoughts with people I have just met because I don't know if they're trustworthy.

- *Are they generally humble or defensive?* If people are unable to sit with their own brokenness and failures, they're not likely to sit well with mine. Of course, everyone gets defensive sometimes. But if somebody has to always be right and can't admit her own faults and struggles, she's less likely to be a good support.

- *Are they encouraging or cutting with their words?* Kindness is such a big deal to me. I come from a big family and totally get sarcastic humor, but I don't open up to people who are generally unkind, judgmental, or cutting toward others.

- *Do they gossip?* If somebody gossips *to* me, I am confident they will gossip *about* me. Again, everybody shares something they shouldn't now and then; I've certainly been guilty of this. If I regularly hear somebody sharing personal or private information about another person, they are not safe to share with.

- *Are they good listeners? Do they make everything about them?* If every conversation turns back to them instead of their being supportive and encouraging listeners, there's a good chance they'll do that when I open up. And if they are always distracted and don't seem to be present for conversations, they probably won't listen well to my pain.

- *Do they have healthy, stable relationships in their lives?* Drama, constant complaints about interpersonal issues, and a lack of long-term relationships can be major red flags. If I'm just getting to know somebody and they are well respected and liked by those close to them (close friends, family members, colleagues), that's a good sign.

Nobody will be perfect at all of these all the time. By paying attention to the people in your life, considering their characters, and especially how they listen and care for others, you can get a pretty good idea of whether or not they're a good place to go for support. As I began to open up to people one by one, I was looking for these traits.

I'd noticed that Alexis was a really good listener and that everybody close to her respected her. My friend Raissa kept confidences and didn't gossip to me about other people. Kelly was humble and asked a lot of good questions instead of assuming she understood or lecturing me about self-harm. Kate, who once joked that sarcasm is her love language, always set that aside when somebody shared their pain, and she earned trust by being consistent in our friendship.

Of course, there were moments when somebody misread the situation and said something that stung a bit. But overall, these traits guided me well. And even when I'm hurt in a relationship with a safe friend, I can talk to them about it, knowing they will be open to feedback and want to mend the relationship.

Somebody Has to Be Willing to Go First

I used to think that being a good leader meant I had it all together. If I could set aside my own aches to serve others, then I could make a difference. I'm sure part of the reason I clung to that belief was that I thought it was terrifying and risky to open up to others about my deepest pain. When I began to let my guard down, I thought I was letting go of what it meant to be seen as a good Christian leader.

I felt like a failure when Alexis found me and pulled me into that laundry room. But she showed me compassion and grace I desperately needed. If that had been the only result of me confessing my relapse, it would have still been worth it for me to let go of that idea of a strong leader as one who doesn't struggle. Before, a handful of people had known about my depression, self-harm, and suicidal thoughts. Now, for the first time in my life, I felt fully loved by an entire community that had seen the sickness that lived in me. When I started talking, I never could have foreseen how opening up would bring such immense healing and support. But my vulnerability wasn't just for me; I was shocked to find how my vulnerability opened the door to help others feel seen and find the courage to fight.

It's become a normal thing for me now, talking about my mental health in small groups, social settings, and workplaces. I still get nervous sometimes; it would be nice to present a more put-together image to those around me. And even as I write this book, there are times I wish I weren't turning my soul inside out for the world to see. But it's gotten much easier to share, and each time, I've found it's worth it to me.

This type of sharing is usually not the same as when you're looking for support from loved ones. I've found that I can talk about depression in a way that is authentic without needing people to respond a certain way. I reserve talking about intimate details of current struggles for close relationships with the safe people in my life. But I will talk more generally about mental health with most people because I know going first might free somebody else. There are a few things I've learned that help me "go first" in sharing my story:

- *Make it casual.* I'll mention in passing that I go to counseling, for example, or that I eat a certain way because it really helps with my anxiety. A lot of times, people say, "Oh, that's cool." But it's not uncommon to hear they deal with panic attacks too or that they just moved to the area and haven't found a good therapist yet. I've never had anybody make fun of me or say anything rude when I've mentioned it.

- *"Speak from scars, not wounds" (at first).*[3] Sometimes, it's easier to talk about times I *have* struggled with depression and things that have helped me through it than to talk about current episodes. For people who I don't know well or who haven't earned some trust, speaking about past experiences helps me create some emotional distance to not feel like I need them to respond especially graciously.
- *Answer questions.* I was hanging out with some coworkers at a conference several years ago when one started talking about a friend of a friend who had attempted suicide. He was genuinely trying to understand why. "I just don't get what could get somebody to that place to do something like that," he said. I took a deep breath and said, "I do. I've actually been there." My coworker looked shocked but then started asking some follow-up questions and eventually thanked me for helping him understand.
- *Look for ways to help.* When friends share that they're having problems in their marriage or are struggling to get through a season of grief, I listen and empathize, then gently ask if they've got a good counselor to talk to. I make sure to share how much of a difference counseling has helped in my relationship with my husband, Micah, and in navigating heartache. I'll even offer to help them find a good therapist and refer mine, if appropriate.
- *Take advantage of dates on the calendar.* May is Mental Health Awareness Month and September is Suicide Prevention and Awareness Month. Organizations like To Write Love on Her Arms often have resources available that make starting a conversation or even sharing something on social media much easier.
- *Use your platform.* I did not start my blog intending to talk about mental illness. I definitely wasn't planning on being the suicide girl. But when I first wrote about depression, even though I had a very small audience at the time, I was overwhelmed at the response. I realized people were desperate—as I had often been—to know they're not alone,

so I started sharing more and more. Eventually, that led to this book. If you're in a position of leadership (whether online or in real life), you might consider speaking up about mental illness. I'm not saying your whole platform needs to be about mental health, but if you have even a handful of people listening to you, a small mention here and there can make a huge difference.

That day, with that group of young women, I learned an important lesson. Once somebody starts to talk about their mental health, it frees others to talk about their own. People are willing to talk about finding counselors, taking meds, and managing their anxiety and depression when they know others will understand them. It's like the *Pay It Forward* principle from the movie: one person impacts a few, and those few impact many. And this is how stigma is erased over time.

When I finally opened up, I learned that it's not enough to just see others talking about their struggles with mental illness. I had seen leaders open up about their struggles, how they got help, took meds, and went to therapy. All of that had opened a door to healing for me. But staying in isolation and refusing to tell my story would have kept me from truly walking through that door. And it certainly would have prevented others from knowing we could walk together on the journey.

I didn't expect to find the support I needed from a community of women who were that much younger than me, whose life experience looked so different. I didn't expect that they would be such a source of strength or that their words of simple care and comfort would be life-sustaining as they demonstrated the love of Christ to me. But I also didn't expect that my "going first" in sharing my story would make room for others to find healing.

Eight

If I Make My Bed in Hell

The room was darkened; if I sat at the edge, nobody could really see my face. I liked it that way. In a room full of church leaders and staff passionately praying for God to move and transform lives, I couldn't connect with their zeal. Tuesday mornings were staff prayer meetings; in a fourteen-thousand-member church, it was easy to disappear in a room of more than a hundred people. I remember the emptiness and the soul ache of that day. Something about being surrounded by such passionate leaders always made it more acute.

Maybe it's because I knew all the "right" things to say and do. I knew all the verses some believed would fill me with joy and "break off a spirit of depression."

For I know the plans I have for you, declares the LORD, plans for welfare and not for evil, to give you a future and a hope. (Jeremiah 29:11)

I can do everything through Christ, who gives me strength. (Philippians 4:13, NLT)

The joy of the LORD is your strength. (Nehemiah 8:10)

The LORD is my shepherd; I shall not want. (Psalm 23:1)

Therefore, if anyone is in Christ, he is a new creation. The old has passed away; behold, the new has come. (2 Corinthians 5:17)

I am fearfully and wonderfully made. (Psalm 139:14)

Rejoice in the Lord always; again I will say, rejoice. (Philippians 4:4)

Years before, I was taught to memorize them, to speak them, to use them to fight back against my emotions. I was taught to "declare Scriptures over myself" and "claim God's promises" to make my life "line up with truth." Even now, I find Pinterest filled with promises to "conquer anxiety" and "defeat depression" simply by reading certain verses.

I knew the Bible says, "The word of God is living and active, sharper than any two-edged sword" (Hebrews 4:12). I knew God said of Scripture, "It shall not return to Me void" (Isaiah 55:11, NKJV), meaning it wouldn't come back without accomplishing everything he sent it to do.

Early on, I simply accepted it all at face value, believing it would work exactly as people told me. But when I spoke those words out, they fell empty from my lips, devoid of the power I'd been taught to expect.

Over time, I discovered that going to the Bible in hope of simply feeling better never worked. It seemed that uttering verses like magic words was a fool's errand. And repeating memorized verses that people told me should fill me with joy . . . it never did.

I didn't know there was something missing.

———

In that dim room, I dutifully opened my Bible to Psalm 139. This passage is the home of some familiar "antidepression" verses, like "I praise you, for I am fearfully and wonderfully made" and the one that says God's thoughts about us outnumber the grains of sand.

Suddenly, the words jumped off the page, shaping an image in my mind: "If I make my bed in hell, behold, You are there" (verse 8, NKJV). I was fetal curled in the black depths of a pit, arms clinging tightly to myself, staring blankly. *If I make my bed in hell . . .* Some translations call it Sheol or the grave. It didn't matter what you call it; I knew that place well, though I'd never imagined it quite like this before. "Making my bed in hell" was more than familiar. What else can you call it when your soul is too weary to try to climb up from that pit?

But what tightened my throat, made me catch my breath, stung my eyes, was the image of Jesus there. In my mind's eye, he sat close behind me, sometimes laying a hand on my shoulder to remind me of his nearness, sometimes just sitting quietly with me.

You are there.

None of the verses people told me to pray and recite have ever worked like the magic words I expected. But when these words came alive, jumped off the page, and embedded themselves deep into my soul? *That's powerful.*

And, dear friend, perhaps you're experiencing this too. Perhaps you have the lists of verses and declarations tucked into your Bible or saved on your phone. Perhaps you've tried to read and pray and connect with God, but it all just seems so empty—or even condemning.

I've been there. And I've learned how to find hope in the Bible when I desperately need it. Here's the secret:

The best Bible verses for hard times are the ones that come alive *to us.*

We don't need magic words or magic wands to make it all better (though I've wished for that so many times). Instead, we need to hear from the mouth of God for ourselves as he breathes into some portion of Scripture until it comes alive to us.

Because, yes, God's Word is living and active. Yes, it is powerful and accomplishes what he sent it to do. I believe that in the core of my being. But if I believe it's God's Word, then he gets to choose what he does with it in my life. I don't get to dictate what he speaks to me or how he uses Scripture to reshape and restore me.

I *can* rest assured that when I open the pages of my Bible, I am meeting with Christ who is the Word made flesh. And that's what I've learned: the Jesus who comes alive in the pages of Scripture has always been Immanuel. That's how he stands out to me, how he speaks to my heart. I've always found hope in verses about him being present in the dark.

So in that prayer meeting with church leaders, he chose the raw, dark imagery of a verse that says, "If I make my bed in hell, behold, You are there" instead of brighter verses like "rejoice in the Lord always" or "be anxious for nothing" (Philippians 4:4, 6, NKJV). That visceral psalm resonated deeply with me because God knows just how much depression, anxiety, and grief can feel hellacious to me.

It's so reassuring that God knows how to speak to us in ways we can understand. We don't need to try so hard to get it right; we just need to show up and trust. And he knew that reminding me he's present in that darkness was more life giving to me in the moment than the hope of getting out of it.

There's a richness and peace that comes when Scripture becomes experiential this way, when we trust God to speak to our deepest needs and longings. If you've never experienced this, or if you've felt like reading the Bible has been all about rules and condemnation, that can change.

Creating New Patterns

Sometimes, it's a battle to read the Bible. We feel like there's something wrong with us for not "getting anything" out of our time reading Scripture. When we see people posting on social media about their picture-perfect quiet times, it seems like it should be so simple. If we're honest about our experiences, we know it's not so easy, especially when wrestling with mental illness. There are legitimate challenges that can get in the way.

One of the biggest obstacles is something called implicit memory. It's our intrinsic capability to learn and remember on an unconscious level. There's a saying that "neurons that fire together wire together"; in other words, all our life experiences create patterns of behavior and emotion in our brains and bodies whether or not we're consciously paying attention. Like the muscle memory that lets you ride a bike after years of not using that skill, these neural patterns can be reactivated, given the right set of circumstances. In fact, the patterns are so automatic that we don't even realize we're remembering something. It just feels completely natural and true.[1]

These patterns and models are really useful because they save energy for us and make things easier. We don't have to consciously think about all the steps to brushing our teeth, for example, once they're embedded in our implicit memory. But just because our brains learn a pattern doesn't make it true, good, or healthy. Painful experiences, lies we believe, trauma, and bad habits also lock implicit memories away inside us. Though we aren't aware of their presence, they touch everything, coloring all our perceptions.

What does this have to do with reading the Bible? Well, those unhealthy and untrue patterns are quick to show themselves when we try to interact with God. If you've experienced someone using Scripture in an abusive, authoritarian, or condemning way, you're bound to filter everything you read through the pain and shame embedded in your implicit memory. If you've experienced harm at the hands of an authority figure, patterns of responses could easily be reactivated. Even the lies and shame of depression can create patterns of belief and behavior that interfere with experiencing Scripture as life giving and hope filled.

This is one of the reasons so many of us can read passages that communicate the tender, affectionate care of God but can't believe they apply to *us*. I've had friends and readers tell me things like "I love Jesus with all my heart, and I know there is no condemnation in Christ, but when I read the Bible, I only see condemnation." I know this feeling intimately because I struggled with it for many, many years. All I saw were the ways I wasn't living up and I wasn't enough. My shame and self-hatred made it nearly impossible to believe anything good I read could apply to me.

But my dear friend and former pastor once told me that we all hear from God "through a dirty filter." This was long before I'd learned the neuroscience behind all this, but it immediately rang true. We must learn to recognize our filters. When we open the

Bible and start to feel shame, condemnation, or as though we're excluded from the goodness of God, we can pause and notice it, reminding ourselves that our painful experiences have lied to us. The kindness and affection of God are still for us, even when we wrestle with such ache and anguish.

Remember, as we discussed in the introduction to this book, our brains can change. While we may never completely erase the old patterns, with practice we can create new ones. Meditation and contemplative prayer are powerful ways to respond to those old patterns. Picking an encouraging, hopeful Bible verse and meditating on it over and over can gradually build new patterns and help us learn to receive the love of God through his Word.

Another major obstacle to connecting with God through Scripture is the cognitive impairment that comes with serious depression. We who wrestle in the dark call it by different names: exhaustion, brain fog, and overwhelm are just a few that come to mind. Experts tell us that depression can change how we think, make it tougher to make decisions—let alone good ones—and impair our ability to focus.[2] Other symptoms of depression that affect our ability to read and learn are fatigue and apathy. In a cruel twist, these symptoms often travel with guilt and shame. We might be exhausted, lack energy, and feel glued to the bed, but that won't stop the crushing guilt for not doing *all the things* we think we should. Some of my readers have shared that they live under constant guilt for "ignoring" God.

There are a few basic principles and perspectives that help me connect with God when I read my Bible. I've also discovered some practices that make it much easier when it's hard to read for any of the myriad reasons that come along with depression.

First, *don't look for a way out, but through.* Reading the Bible doesn't change our immediate circumstances. It doesn't instantly fix what's going on in our brains and bodies. On some level, we know that, but I've often thought, *God, I'm reading the Bible and doing everything right, so why don't you fix this?*

God is often more concerned with helping us walk through suffering with him than immediately delivering us from it. (I know, this can be so frustrating!) Sometimes, we do have to go *through* "the Valley of Weeping" the Bible talks about (Psalm 84:6, NLT). Still, Scripture is overflowing with messages of comfort and hope for those of us walking through the dark. We may need to let go of the idea that we can fix our problems in order to receive the comfort we need.

Second, *don't look for answers, but for Immanuel*. This is tough because our Western post-Enlightenment society has taught us to seek logical explanations for everything. The apologetics movement, though helpful in many ways, has often reduced the rich mystery of Christ as the Word made flesh to a series of explanations and answers. And in the confusion of depression, we desperately want to make sense of things. We want answers for why we feel this way and how to stop it so we can fix it or prevent it.

As I've learned to reject a bankrupt view of Scripture that reduces it to rules and formulas and answers, I've found beauty, hope, and life. I've learned I won't find answers for why I hurt aside from the simple reality that our world is broken. Sometimes people make terrible choices simply because we have the freedom to make decisions and a loving God who, despite its repeatedly breaking his heart, refuses to violate our free will. Sometimes we're deeply hurt by those choices, or by illness, or by disastrous circumstances. And we may never have answers in our lifetimes.

But we *will* always have Immanuel, our God with Us. So, instead of looking for answers, we must learn to look for the God who sees, who stays, who refuses to leave. We look for parts of the Bible that remind us God won't bail on us, abandon us, or forsake us.

Third, *remember you're always filtering*. When I notice myself thinking *that doesn't apply to me*, I remind myself that I'm perceiving what I read through implicit memory and old pain. That gives me the mental space to step back and remember that even if the kindness of God doesn't *feel* true at the moment, it still is. (By the way, this is a helpful practice that applies to every relationship and interaction, not just our relationship with God and Scripture.)

Fourth, *know God can talk to you in a way you understand*. My former pastor taught me this one as well, and I've found it to be breathtakingly true. When I feel bad that I'm not getting any great revelations from my quiet time, I remember that it's not up to me to make God speak or for something to jump off the page. God knows how we're made and what we really need. He's kind enough to speak hope in a way I can receive it. My only job is to show up and be open.

Once we make those perspective shifts, there are some very practical things we can do to make it easier to connect with God.

Lower your standards. If you're hard on yourself or feel guilty about not reading the Bible, give yourself some grace. Don't try to read long passages or do deep study. Don't try to keep up perfectly with a reading plan every day (unless the rhythm and consistency feels good and guilt-free to you).

Spending time with God is not an obligation and it doesn't make him love you more. It's something that is supposed to be life giving and encouraging, not something riddled with guilt for not being good enough. And here's the truth: God knows you have a mental illness that makes it really stinking tough to focus and read. So he's not surprised or disappointed when you struggle.

I've learned to set very low microcommitment standards when I'm struggling. For long seasons when I battled depression, I kept my Bible by my bed and read just a verse or two from the Psalms before I turned out the light. That's it. Sometimes I would also jot down anything that stuck out to me or journal about questions I had. The low expectations make it less likely to trigger shame, so it's easier to keep reading. When I feel up to it, I read more. But a tiny bit of hope every day is way better than trying to spend an hour reading my Bible, feeling discouraged, and then not picking it up again for two weeks.

Mix it up. If it's hard to read the Bible because of apathy, brain fog, or focus problems, there are lots of other great ways to interact with Scripture. The YouVersion Bible app will read to you while you lie in bed or even multitask. During one season when I struggled with depression *and* busyness, I found audio devotionals to listen to during my commute.

Read a story from a children's Bible, put one key verse on your lock screen and read it every day, or sign up for an email or app-based devotional that sets reminders for you. There are also incredible animated videos from BibleProject on YouTube that explore tons of topics and are a great way to still grow in your understanding of God's Word when it's hard to read.

Engage with hope, encouragement, and lament. We have so much in common with those whose stories are recorded in the Bible because their lives weren't perfect. People lost children, lost their homes, lost their loved ones. People were kidnapped and taken into slavery, mistreated because of their gender or ethnicity, forced to flee as refugees, and experienced genocide. And they talked about it.

I think our instinct is often to look for hope-filled, encouraging verses that might help us feel better. There is great value in that. But seeing Jesus grieve and weep, reading the raw expressions of anguish in Lamentations, and connecting with the depths of the psalmists' despair can be cathartic and healing as we remember we aren't alone.

Choose stories, poems, and songs. Listen, friend, I'm a nerd. I love digging deep into obscure stuff in the Bible, but even I won't try to read dense passages when I'm struggling to focus. Leave the theology-heavy passages or long lists of Old Testament laws for another time. We're naturally wired to connect with stories, so choose familiar, comforting stories that reveal beautiful things about the character and kindness of God.

Biblical poetry covers the full spectrum of human emotion. You'll find everything from heartbroken laments to angry rants, from joyful praise to accusations against God. You can find a psalm for just about any mood or commiserate with Job's pain. Plus, the creative, rhythmic, and symbolic aspects of poetry activate different parts of our brains and connect to emotional states and implicit memory in ways that can be restorative and healing.[3]

Always come back to Jesus. This never fails me. When I see shame, condemnation, or guilt in the pages of Scripture, I come back to the Gospels and back to Jesus. Because he rebuked Pharisees for putting impossible religious burdens on people (Matthew 23:4). He told good, churchgoing people they had no right to punish a woman caught in adultery and told her he wouldn't condemn her either

(John 8:1–11). Jesus *is* the Word made flesh and God with Us. He's the perfect expression of the love, mercy, and justice of God. Over and over, returning to Jesus reminds me that I am seen, known, and loved by God.

Try lectio divina. Lectio divina is Latin for "divine reading" and it's a simple, meditative way of engaging with Scripture through a four-step process. This ancient method originated before the invention of the printing press, in a time when most people didn't have access to their own Bibles. The easy process is a great complement to contemplative prayer and works well when you can't focus long enough to read long passages.

- *Lectio* means reading and consists of slowly reading a short passage of Scripture while paying attention to what stands out most to you.
- *Meditatio* means reflecting on the passage. Read the parts that stuck out again, reflecting on them and listening for what God might speak to you. Take your time here.
- *Oratio* means praying the passage. Talk to God about what stuck out, ask him to make it real to you, or ask what he wants to show you.
- *Contemplatio* means simply resting in the love of God and the truth revealed to you through this passage.

Go deeper. In the hardest moments, what matters most is that we can connect with God in his Word. But when we can on our better days, it's important to dig deeper into Bible study. This is how I've established a foundation of confidence in the character of God.

There's another simple, popular method of Bible study that's perfect for beginners called SOAP (for Scripture, Observation, Application, and Prayer). While lectio divina is contemplative, SOAP focuses on study. When you read a passage of Scripture, jot it down. Then, note any observations (what sticks out to you) and how you think it might apply to your life. Then take a few moments to talk to God about it in prayer.[4] To gain a deeper understanding, look at different Bible versions, search for online commentaries, and look at translations of the original Greek and Hebrew words.[5]

I also love to search "historical context of (whatever verse I'm looking at)" because the Bible was written a long time ago in several different cultures. It's hugely helpful to understand those cultural differences because otherwise we can misunderstand the significance of what we're reading. BibleProject on YouTube is great for learning about context and the big picture of what we're reading.

Digging deeper in this way is a great part of our long-term walk with God, but it may not be feasible on dark days when you can barely focus. Give yourself grace on the days when you need it and just focus on trying to connect with God's love and hope. There will be time for the rest of it on brighter days.

There is power in speaking truth to the lies that come with severe mental illness, and we will look at that in a future chapter. But what I learned in that dark room is that sometimes it's much more powerful to sit with Scripture and let the Holy Spirit make something come alive for me.

For years, I didn't understand the Bible. Whenever I tried to read Scripture, I couldn't focus and I filtered my perceptions of God through painful circumstances and deep wounds. I didn't *really* believe God loved me because I couldn't connect with what I read. No matter what the words on the page said, they couldn't *really* have applied to me.

These days, I find hope and love when I open Scripture. Most of all, I connect with God. He's become my comforter, my strength, my very dearest friend. But it took a while to get there. It's okay if it takes a little while for you too. I promise you, it's worth the journey.

Let it be a process, my friend. Let go of some of the pressure. Today, give yourself permission to not read and recite the "right" verses. Give yourself permission to show up, honest and raw and vulnerable, and let God speak to you with kindness through his Word.

Nine

The Darkness May Always Be There

After years of battling severe depression and suicidal thoughts, I was weary. This particular season of depression was especially exhausting, with its fast-paced schedule and my overly full calendar.

I sat at a stoplight, trembling with anxiety's rattle and hum. The sky was bleak with charcoal clouds that seemed to mirror my soul. The familiar fog of depression had rolled in, and I was weary of the struggle. It was exhausting: wrestling to be whole, never shaking the bone-deep loneliness. The fog formed a dense wall, hedging me into isolation. Most days, it seemed nobody, not even God, could break through.

There's an excruciating physicality to mental illness that's rarely acknowledged. But this pain was nothing new. I couldn't remember a time before depression's waves rolled through my body. I'd grown accustomed to smiling, saying I was just tired, doing my best to show up for my commitments while my chest burned and my body felt like lead.

Still, the worst part was the way secret questions carved out my insides. *God, are you there? Why can't I be different? Why won't you fix me? I know you can.*

It wasn't just the questions but the story I believed underneath them: *God doesn't want this mess and neither does anyone else.* And even deeper still was the hidden belief that if I didn't someday get better, I wasn't enough. If I didn't someday overcome, I wasn't worthy.

By now, I knew God loved me. But what if there was a time

limit on his grace and the clock was running out? What if he got tired of me dealing with these same struggles? I still believed some of the things I'd been told over the years, that "depression is so self-focused" and maybe if I wasn't so selfish, I'd get better. Maybe I just needed to choose joy, as I'd been told for so long.

But in my mind, *choose joy* sounded an awful lot like *snap out of it.* Those words left my skin flushed hot and nausea rising in my throat. I'd tried, *so hard,* and I just couldn't figure it out. I just kept failing. Countless begging prayers with all the faith I could muster hadn't changed the ache inside. Years of spending every free moment in ministry, serving and caring without rest, hadn't filled the gaping void.

I'd found friends who loved and accepted me despite the darkness. I'd learned that opening up about depression wasn't only healing for me but let others know they could be honest too. But there were still things I didn't understand.

Would I ever get better? Would I always be sick? I was still single, much longer than I'd hoped; would anybody ever want me? Or was I too broken to share my life with another person?

How could I keep doing this?

I hid my big questions and unkempt prayers until I could let out the mess, alone in my car. That old Taurus became a safe place to me, a sanctuary in a busy season when I found little time for myself. Between the busyness and the fatigue, my car had grown as messy as my soul felt. Empty paper cups rolled on the floorboards. Clothes were strewn over boxes of books and trinkets—I was always moving, always going here to there. Despite the clutter, that old car was my safe place. There was no need to smile, no show to put on. Nobody to hear or judge.

I was running ministry errands that day, grateful for a reprieve from interaction in the offices. My heart raced with a sinking question: *What if I never get better?* Shame seared my flushed skin. *Nobody wants this. How do I live like this forever?*

There at the stoplight, my body trembled as the gray and weight and cloud pressed in. My thoughts spiraled and buzzed. The bony hand of anxiety started to close around my throat, and my breath became shallow, tight.

On the edge of despair, I heard a gentle whisper in my heart: *The darkness may always be there, but I will always be there in the darkness.*

My mouth gaped open, eyes wide and welling with tears. But it wasn't sorrow. It was hope, bittersweet, shocking hope. To some, it might have sounded like a death sentence. But not to me. It was a first-time promise of life. That whisper in my heart, *The darkness may always be there,* told me to stop fighting to fix myself through my own efforts.

Stop burying the pain.

Stop hiding the melancholy that lives inside; stop trying so hard to make it go away. It's okay that it's there, and it's okay that it's so hard. It's okay to face bravely into it, to let go of denial and learn to live with it for the long term.

The second half of that whisper was sweeter still. *I will always be there in the darkness.* It shook my soul like tectonic plates shifting, foundations rearranged. I reeled from the shock of realization and remembrance that God isn't disappointed in me.

There's no countdown clock on grace, no limit on his love. He's not tapping his foot and looking at his watch, impatient for me to get it together. He sits with me in the confusing, aching darkness. The rattle and hum quieted, vibrations and tension slowly fading. I remembered that verse from Psalm 139 that I'd read months before: *If I make my bed in hell, you're there.* The heaviness in my chest lifted as I drew a deep breath.

Years ago, I heard someone say *the voice of God is always wiser and kinder than our own.* I think that's how I recognized those words as coming from him because I never would have said them to myself. Those words released so much guilt and fear. They pledged that I'm not so profoundly screwed up that the God of the universe would ever back away. He isn't afraid of my depression. He doesn't shrink from the darkness. And if he can accept me like this for the rest of my days on earth, I can learn to accept myself too.

———

Maybe, like me, you're weary of fighting and trying to push back the depression. Maybe you've spent countless hours asking why God won't fix you or take away the pain.

Acceptance can be a multilayered process, and it was for me. For the past year, I'd been coming to terms with the reality that I deal with depression, but that day in my car was another layer of coming to terms with what it meant that I might *always* have depression. It was a powerful turning point for me. Now, like Paul, I have found that when God doesn't take away the "thorn in the flesh," his grace is still more than enough for me, even in the pain of depression (2 Corinthians 12:7–9).

I don't know why it seems like some people get answers to their prayers for healing and transformation and some don't. But in my life, I've experienced this wild paradox: when I started to accept that I may have a mental illness for the rest of my life, it became much less painful. While it may sound like despair or giving up to say this is probably what the rest of my life will be like, it can actually be a life-giving, hopeful perspective.

Here's why.

Instead of spending so much energy beating myself up for something that's outside my control, I can direct that energy to learning how to live well despite the mental illness. Instead of feeling like I struggle because I'm a bad Christian or have a moral failing, I can let go of shame and know that my illness is just as legitimate as diabetes or asthma or anything else. Instead of believing God is going to get tired of me being so "selfish," I can rest in the promises that he's not going to bail on me in the midst of my pain.

Depression isn't my fault, and it's not yours either. It's the complicated result of a ton of factors, and it's not something I can wish or pray away. Instead, it's part of my life. For me, acceptance started with a simple realization: *even if the darkness is there forever, God will be with me in the darkness.*

God isn't upset, disappointed, or even mildly irritated with your struggles, my friend. And even if you never fully "get over" mental illness, God is with you. His grace is there to help carry you through the hardest moments. And he wants to help make your life rich and beautiful *even with* depression.

It's not either-or. You are not disqualified from the abundant, more-than-enough, joyful life Jesus promised just because your brain and body are sick. There is a path to wellness that's not getting over this but going through it. And we're going on that journey together.

This Is Hard—and Incredibly Normal

Mental illness is painful, and we so often just want it to stop. We don't want to believe it may stay with us for the long term, so it's tempting to reject that reality. When I was ready to move past denial, I had started by accepting that depression played some role in my life; but now, I had to accept it was a *chronic* part of my life. For me, that acceptance started with the realization that God wouldn't abandon me in the darkness, even if it never leaves me. But it would have been so helpful to me to understand how common it is for depression to be a recurrent or even lifelong condition.

Half of all chronic mental illness starts before the age of fourteen and three-quarters before the age of twenty-four, and those who, like me, experience an early onset of mental illness are especially likely to live with it their whole lives.[1] The *Diagnostic and Statistical Manual of Mental Disorders* tells us that major depressive disorder is a recurrent disease in most cases, meaning it goes into remission before eventually coming back. There's also a chronic form of depression called persistent depressive disorder (also called dysthymia or chronic major depressive disorder) that can be diagnosed when an episode lasts more than two years in adults or one year in children or teens. And the presence of other mental health challenges—anxiety, unresolved childhood trauma, or personality disorders, for example—increases the likelihood of chronic or recurrent depression.[2]

One study suggested that at least 50 percent of people who have one major depressive episode will go on to have another; 80 percent of those who have experienced two or more episodes will have at least one more recurrence.[3] More recent research has indicated that more than 85 percent of patients will experience a recurrence within ten years of their first episode, and about half will have one within six months of going into remission if their treatment is discontinued.[4]

If this is your first dance with the darkness, all these statistics may be frightening. If you've lived with this for a while, they may seem discouraging. But what if they mean there's nothing wrong with you for not getting over it so easily? What if they mean it's not all in your head, you're not failing, and there's help available to you? As I read these statistics, my heart breathed a sigh of relief. *Oh, this is normal.* Sometimes I still need that reminder. This is hard, and also incredibly normal.

The other reason I see hope in these statistics is that it means mental illness—particularly chronic mental illness—is well studied. Researchers are committed to understanding and finding better treatments for this thing that causes so much suffering. After all, neuropsychiatric disorders (the category that includes mental illness and neurological problems) are the leading cause of disability in the United States.[5] They not only cause great suffering but also massive economic impacts to the tune of hundreds of billions of dollars lost annually.[6] While I know many scientists and researchers are motivated by altruistic reasons to find solutions, it certainly doesn't hurt that it's in the best interest of corporations and governments to support and fund research into mental health.

What Now?

We're slowly becoming more accustomed to talking about depression and anxiety in the church. I've started hearing more sermons and faith-based podcasts that mention mental health issues, seeing posts on social media, and noticing lots of Christian books about anxiety. Sadly, much of this openness is being fueled by high-profile suicides of pastors and their family members over the past few years. These tragedies are forcing us to confront the reality of mental illness and have much-needed conversations.

Unfortunately, we're still not very comfortable with talking about what it means to live with a lifelong disorder. It's easier to acknowledge situational depression, perhaps linked to grief or postpartum hormonal changes. But for many, severe depression is a chronic illness that requires a paradigm shift and a new level of acceptance. As we come face to face with the possibility that we may deal with severe depression or suicidal thoughts for the rest of our lives, we must be prepared for two things.

First, we must shift our mindsets. Instead of just looking for ways to deal with the current struggles, we must play the long game with our mental health, recognizing the choices we can make to set ourselves up for better health. We'll learn to slow down, set boundaries, work with doctors and mental health professionals, and implement habits that set us up to truly live well for the long term.

Second, we need to know that true faith means trusting God even when he doesn't change our circumstances. When we accept that God may never choose to heal us, some well-meaning Christians might take that to mean we've lost faith or given up on God. In those moments, I remind myself that my brothers and sisters really want what they believe to be the best for me and they believe that means being cured. I get that, and I would be thrilled if that's what God did for me. And I understand why people cling to this belief—it's simpler and easier than wrestling with a good God who allows suffering and doesn't always rescue us from it.

But the truth is that my faith—and perhaps yours as well—has been forged in the fires of pain. Those of us who can say, with Paul, that the grace and love of God is enough even when we continue to suffer know something about faith that we just can't learn by overcoming everything. We don't have to be healed to trust him. Our hope rests on his character, who he's proved himself to be time and again through presence in the midst of pain.

Rest assured, my friend, that true, healthy acceptance of chronic illness requires faith that God will walk with us through the struggle for as long as it takes. This is the faith of Job, who said of God, "Though he slay me, I will hope in him" even as he continued to lament and express his pain (Job 13:15). It doesn't always make sense to those who haven't walked through the fire, but it does to us.

We need not be ashamed because we know whom we have believed (2 Timothy 1:12). God is with us. He isn't leaving. He isn't giving up. If the darkness will always be here, so will God. He'll sit in its midst with us, holding our sometimes-desperate, flailing hearts. We won't be alone. Maybe that's all we need to know to get through.

Ten

Living with a Limp

I saw the Tahoe a split second before it barreled into me. It was a beautiful spring day, and I was out on a run. The central Oregon skies were clear and blue, and the air was just crisp enough to keep me moving. I'd stopped at an intersection, waited for the signal to alert me to cross, and glanced both ways before I took two or three steps into the crosswalk. I noticed the glint of sunlight off the shiny hood and felt my heart jump hard against my ribs. People tell me I screamed, but I don't remember it.

Fifty-eight-hundred pounds of SUV threw me like a rag doll before I landed in a crumpled heap on the asphalt. The next thing I knew, I was sitting on a curb, people circling and chattering. I was shaking inside, but I forced myself to smile. "I'm fine."

Maybe I was just saying it to convince myself. *I'm okay. I don't live far. I can walk home. I'm fine. Everything is fine.* The lady who hit me was crying. People wanted to call 911. *I'm fine,* I kept insisting. *I'm fine.*

Adrenaline is a powerful enough drug that for a while I believed myself. Someone finally talked me into going to the emergency room and getting checked out. And it turns out, I did seem fine, just a little banged up: no broken bones, no obvious internal injuries, and not much pain for the first few hours.

Of course, adrenaline eventually wears off, and I soon realized what people mean when they say, "I feel like I got hit by a truck." Muscles I didn't know existed ached and swelled. I was nauseous, my head pounded, and I could barely move. Still, I refused to take time off work because it was a busy season. I kept showing up to ministry events, sometimes on little sleep. I squeezed in doctor appointments, three sessions of physical therapy per week, and continued to write sermons and lead a youth group.

It never occurred to me to slow down, though my body screamed for it. Muscles would freeze and lock when I finally sat down, and I sometimes found myself stuck, unable to rise from my chair or when I lay down to stretch. Nerves burned in my arms, my legs, my face, as though an unseen fire raged; nothing seemed to put it out.

The symptoms from my head injury didn't show up for weeks, but when they did, they were brutal. I couldn't remember my Social Security number or things I'd just said. Black spots danced across my vision, I kept dropping things, and I couldn't read more than a short sentence. Conversations that used to be easy for me to follow became frustrating and tear inducing. I felt humiliated that I couldn't understand things as easily as I always had and that I had to keep asking for clarification. A few appointments with a neurologist and an MRI to rule out a brain hemorrhage left me diagnosed with post-concussive syndrome and on mandatory "brain rest" for several weeks.

I'd never heard of such a thing, but it basically meant that I couldn't work, couldn't read, and couldn't even watch much TV for two weeks. I took a lot of naps and went to physical therapy. I was forced to slow down. My body and brain needed time to heal. Around the same time, as weeks stretched into months and my other injuries weren't healing well, a doctor told me it would have been better if my body had broken instead of stretching.

I discovered I have something called hypermobility syndrome: my joints stretch too far. Broken bones heal, my doctor said, and the break absorbs some of the force of the injury. But soft tissue can stretch only so far before there's irreparable damage. The flexibility that had always been my strength suddenly became a liability.

That was true in my life too. The way I kept moving, kept saying yes, kept "being flexible" seemed like a benefit. I thought I was strong and capable. But really, that overflexibility allowed me to experience more pain and more damage as I pushed myself beyond what should have been the breaking point.

The experience of being hit by an SUV lasted only moments and left me with a body that was forever altered by injuries and pain. And the lesson I didn't learn from getting hit by an SUV came back to me after a bad relapse with self-harm and suicidal thoughts: I needed to slow down. I had to stop pretending I was fine and learn to live with my limp.

Learning to Limp

I am not the first person to desperately need this lesson. There's this wild story from Genesis that illustrates it perfectly:

> And Jacob was left alone. And a man wrestled with him until the breaking of the day. When the man saw that he did not prevail against Jacob, he touched his hip socket, and Jacob's hip was put out of joint as he wrestled with him. Then he said, "Let me go, for the day has broken." But Jacob said, "I will not let you go unless you bless me." And he said to him, "What is your name?" And he said, "Jacob." Then he said, "Your name shall no longer be called Jacob, but Israel, for you have striven with God and with men, and have prevailed." Then Jacob asked him, "Please tell me your name." But he said, "Why is it that you ask my name?" And there he blessed him. So Jacob called the name of the place Peniel, saying, "For I have seen God face to face, and yet my life has been delivered." The sun rose upon him as he passed [Peniel], limping because of his hip. (Genesis 32:24–31)

There's some debate on the identity of the being who wrestled with Jacob. We don't know for sure whether it was an angel or perhaps the preincarnate Christ. But Jacob said that he had seen God face to face, so I tend to take him at his word and believe it was Christ who wrestled with Jacob through the long dark night.

I don't know if that detail matters, really, aside from the fact that we can often feel like we're wrestling God. For our purposes, the point is that Jacob refused to give up, despite the fact that he was in pain. The word used in Hebrew doesn't just mean to "prevail" or "overcome," but to "endure."[1]

Sometimes, it seems impossible to hold on in the darkness, doesn't it? Sometimes it seems that day will never dawn, we will never take hold of any blessing, and all that lies ahead is endless midnight. Despite the confusion and pain, Jacob endured. He hung on when it didn't make sense, until he emerged from that fight with two things: a new name and a new limp.

The name would forever be a reminder: he had wrestled with God and overcome. He had endured one of the hardest fights of his life. And I wonder if, whenever his hip ached and he limped, the sound of his new name reminded him that he had endured before and could endure again.

In my experience, a limp impacts so much of my life. But it doesn't prevent me from living it. My accident left me with several lasting injuries, and on occasion, the pain causes me to limp. It's an impairment that forces me to slow down, to adapt, to move in different ways, but it's not paralysis. I can still walk, though it may be slow and difficult at times. Sometimes, I really need to rest.

This is true of my mental health too. For me and many others, depression is a chronic illness. I have good days and bad, times when I can keep pace and others when my limp is more prominent. Like Jacob, I've had to learn to adjust, to slow down, to listen to my own needs instead of trying to meet the expectations of everyone around me.

The Science of Stress

One of my biggest lessons in living with my limp has been learning to manage stress. It seemed almost too simple; for a lot of years, I thought busy schedules and constant activity were the norm and had little to do with the clouds that followed me around. But as I learned what it meant to live with lifelong depression, it became obvious that one of the first things I needed to do was learn to slow down.

Stress is what happens when we experience undue burdens on our resources.[2] When we experience stressful situations, our bodies release a cascade of hormones that create real physiological changes designed to help us respond. Adrenaline, cortisol, and other hormones rush through our systems, giving us the energy we need to fight for our lives or run to safety. This is the well-known "fight-or-flight response."[3]

These physiological changes aren't intended to last very long. Once the threat is past, our bodies are supposed to return to a state of equilibrium as stress hormones dissipate. When we are consistently overscheduled and overburdened by stress, that cascade of hormones becomes toxic as it overwhelms our bodies and brains. Chronic stress increases our chances of developing mental illnesses and are known to worsen symptoms of depression and anxiety.[4]

Of course, it's not just a busy schedule that causes problems. Any chronic stress has a negative effect over time, and society is growing increasingly stressful. As technology advances, expectations of being constantly available and endlessly productive increase.

As I write this, we are in the midst of the global COVID-19 pandemic and widespread protests against racial injustice. People are struggling financially, facing uncertainty, and fighting for justice and dignity. Anxiety over unemployment and health is the highest it has been in my lifetime. And while many of us are just waking up to the reality of the collective trauma, people of color in the United States have been living under the toxic stress of an oppressive society for centuries. It's no wonder so many of us in this nation deal with depression and anxiety.

Of course, I say this from a place of privilege. Sure, I don't come from money, and I know what it's like to barely make ends meet, to fear overdraft fees, and to pick up extra shifts to try to cover bills. But I can still recognize that as a white woman, I've faced fewer obstacles than many on my road to a mentally healthy life. For example, men of all races are less likely to receive mental health treatment than women,[5] while Black and Hispanic people access mental health services about half as much as white people in the United States.[6] Gender-based stigma, cultural differences, poverty, lack of education, and structural inequalities all make it more difficult to reduce stress and get desperately needed mental health care.

In light of all this, it's important to recognize that some stressful situations don't have easy answers; they won't be resolved overnight. It's easy to say "just reduce your stress" when we're financially secure, healthy, and don't live with severe trauma or systemic oppression. While these larger societal issues create stress on a macro level for many people, we can still look at ways to reduce stress on a micro level in our lives. For me, one of the first ones was learning to carve out pockets of time to stop performing and just *be*. At first, this meant taking a few minutes at the end of a long day to do something I enjoyed. Sometimes, I'd sketch for a few minutes or work on a creative project. I've found it's important to make sure I'm not constantly staring at a screen, so art and craft projects have been helpful for me. Making time to get outside, even to see the sun for just ten minutes, makes a huge difference. And meditation has been shown over and over to reduce stress and anxiety,[7] so I try to include some quiet time just focusing on my breath each day. (For more practical tips on stress reduction, see chapter 15, on self-care.)

But learning to live with my limp has required me to do much more than justify little pockets of time doing something relaxing. I've had to take a hard look at my need to perform, overcommit, and constantly prove my worth through work. I've learned that I need a slower pace to life than I once believed. Instead of saying yes to every opportunity to serve or spend time with people, I have had to learn to pay attention to my stress levels and how much margin I have in my life before committing.

There is no shame in rationing energy, considering carefully, and saving our commitments for things we know we can handle without causing harm to ourselves. There's no shame in acknowledging the trade-offs and choosing wisely. Sometimes the house may not be as clean as I'd like. Sometimes we may not be able to prioritize serving at church or volunteering in the community. Sometimes we say yes to something we really want to do, knowing we may set aside some other commitments for a season. You're not a bad person for prioritizing your own well-being. It's okay to listen when your whole being is crying out for a slower pace.

Listening to Your Limp

Some interpret Jacob's injury as affecting his sciatic nerve.[8] This could have left him with burning, numbness, and tingling along the longest nerve in his body, from his lower back and down his leg. We call this sciatica, and it's one of the lingering sources of pain I have from my accident. It's interesting that the pain can come and go, flare up and settle down. Sometimes, it's utterly debilitating. Others, it doesn't really impact my life much.

I don't know if this was really Jacob's injury, but mental illness can follow a similar pattern. Severe depression can come in waves, sometimes heavy and hard ones. Other times, it's a manageable, dull ache or even fades completely for a season. My experiences with chronic pain have taught me that I need to listen to my body and take it easy when I first notice signs of pain. I need to start doing the things that will strengthen and support my body while not demanding it to push through and endure worsening pain.

We have to do this with our mental health. We need to learn to set boundaries, to say no, to notice the first signs of depression flaring up and act accordingly. We can learn to live well with our limps.

Even today, my limp doesn't let me forget it's there. When stress compounds—as when a pandemic, a devastating tornado in my community, and financial uncertainty hit all at once—I more acutely feel the anxiety, the illogical fear, the remnants of trauma, and the shadows of despair. I've tried to find rhythms to keep moving in the midst of uncertainty. But the truth is, upheaval in my life makes my limp more prominent.

I've learned the best way to move through seasons of stress like this is to listen more closely to my body. I pay attention to the emotional signals it gives me: my heart rate, the depth of my breathing, the tension in the back of my neck, my nervous stomach. It's telling me to slow down, to relax a little, and to breathe deeply. So I'm listening. I'm choosing not to push through.

Sure, I might be able to put pressure on myself to pull it together and make things happen and be super productive now. And some seasons do call for us to press through and make things happen. But I also know that my soul, my body, and my mind will all pay for it later. The extra burden of stress will leave me with flared-up symptoms of depression, anxiety, and even physical pain. Taking it easy, listening to my limp, and not pushing it now means that I'll feel like I'm back on level ground all the sooner.

It Doesn't Have to Define You

There's a small white frame that sits on my bookshelf. It holds some patterned paper with a handwritten note and a new name: *She Who Won the Struggle at Dawn.* That name was given to me by a friend who walked alongside me while I learned to live with my limp.

"You've been wrestling and fighting, just like Jacob," she said, "but the answer may not have been what you would have hoped. Instead, you've been left with a limp. So you've had to come to terms with this, to accept your limp, and somehow still refuse to let it define you."

If we are to limp for the rest of our lives, we may never run or walk like others. We will certainly need to treat our bodies and souls with special care if we are to live healthy, thriving lives. Jacob's limp would have impacted nearly everything he did for the rest of his life—walking, working, sitting, if he ever rode mules or horses. He probably needed to rest more than others. There were probably times that he couldn't work because of the pain. There might have been times when he asked why this was the cost of the blessing, after a night that was already long and painful because of the fight.

But he won. He won the struggle at dawn. Winning didn't mean he pinned the Christ-man he wrestled. It meant he didn't give up, even through immense pain. It meant he hung on long enough to be renamed, blessed, and called one who struggles and wins.

Living with a limp may mean that we're going to be well accustomed to this brutal darkness. But it also means that we can learn to find peace in clinging to Christ even in the pain, even when we feel like we're being devoured from the inside out. It means taking good care of our bodies and souls, battling to believe the sun is still there, tucked away behind the clouds, even when we can't see it.

That white picture frame still sits on my bookshelf, reminding me of what a friend saw in me: Someone who can win the struggle. Someone who can live with a limp, but not be defined by it.

Right now, I wish I could look straight at you and speak those same words over you: you are one who wins the struggle at dawn. My dear friend, I know how this aches, how it's hard to just keep breathing sometimes. But I believe you are one who can endure, clinging to God in the midst of the painful, dark night. And when this night season is over, even if there are remnants left in the form of a limp, you can still do this. You can live with your limp; it doesn't have to define you.

Part Three

THRIVING

Eleven

Sit in the Dark

Everything seemed to be going well. I had just moved to Nash-ville, was working a job I adored, and felt full of hope for a bright future. I was the happiest I had ever been. That's probably why I was so surprised when I sensed an invitation to sit in the dark.

In this bright season, I'd started working as a residential assistant in a faith-based therapeutic facility for young women. The residents were well acquainted with the darkness; many lived with mental illnesses and unresolved trauma. It was an incredible privilege to walk alongside these young women. I found joy and purpose working in a healing and redemptive environment, sharing my struggles with depression, suicide, and self-harm, as well as ways I'd learned to navigate the darkness.

The schedule was intense: I worked a sixty-four-hour shift each weekend, from Friday afternoon to Monday morning. During that time, I stayed on-site, helping keep the home running smoothly, mediating conflict, handling first aid, and breathing with residents through panic attacks. Sometimes staff members had to sit up late with residents on suicide watch; other times, we had medical emergencies in the middle of the night.

It wasn't uncommon to get too little sleep, but I believed I could recover well enough during the long stretches between shifts that I'd be able to handle it. And despite the intensity, it was still the most fulfilling job I'd ever had as I watched lives transform right before me.

Even so, many of these young women were working through the aftermath of serious hurt. In my role as a mentor and support to them, I found myself listening to story after story of severe trauma. While I loved my job, exposure to these stories reminded me of some of my own painful experiences. I pushed them down, tried to shake them off, and focused on the work before me.

With all of this, of course, I was weary. But what first seemed like just the tiring transition of the schedule and the type of work developed into an extended, unexplained illness when I suddenly fell ill for two months with something like mono or the flu. When the physical weakness and nausea subsided, the soul-deep weariness remained. I didn't notice at first that the depression was returning. Then a friend I hadn't seen in a while asked what I was excited about, and the only thing that came to mind was sleep. *Huh,* I thought, *that's not a good sign.*

Not long after that, I began to have panic attacks at work and found myself hiding in the meds room to take deep breaths as my heart beat wildly inside. I'd lean against the door, slide to the ground, and try to feel steady again. Next came the nightmares; dark thoughts of self-harm and suicide soon followed.

When the old horror films started playing in my head, filling my mind with countless ways to hurt myself, I knew it was time to get help. Driving on the highway, cutting up vegetables for lunch, or seeing any object that could be used as a weapon gave my mind the opportunity to come up with new self-harm scenarios. Talking with struggling residents or bandaging their self-harm wounds started to feel like a minefield as I navigated my own triggers.

As the fog of depression rolled in again, as the color and joy started to drain out of my life, I sensed an invitation to truly partner with God in my healing process with a simple phrase: *sit in the dark.* It came to me when I was journaling, processing the strange dichotomy of the darkness showing up when my life had never been better. I looked at what I wrote and took that strange, quiet thought to be the voice of God. It's sometimes tough to know when the still, small voice is from the Spirit and not my own mind, but the way I wanted to resist and keep up the status quo was a clue to me. *My life is good,* I argued. *I'll get over this. Why should I sit in the dark?*

I was terrified to engage the ghosts that haunted beneath the surface of my depression. Even as I'd learned to accept mental illness as part of my life, my instinct was still to run for the light. I refused to let my eyes adjust to the shadows so I could see what lingered there. In a church culture that taught me to claim victory over the darkness, it almost seemed heretical to sit with it, even for a short time. *I want this to be simple. I want to push through it and call it done for this round,* I wrote in my journal that day.

But I knew there was more to it. There were painful experiences and beliefs I hadn't dealt with, soul holes that needed filling, monsters that howled around the sides of consciousness. I knew that when the young women I worked with shared their brokenness with me, I spoke hope and truth over them that I couldn't claim for myself.

I told them they were doing good work in therapy and in community, that it was important that they deal with the traumatic memories and the lies they believed about themselves. But I privately clung to the American dream model of healing, the pull-yourself-up-by-your-bootstraps, be-strong-and-capable way of getting better.

4/8/16

When do you sit in the darkness?
When do you run to the light?
My self-sufficient streak tells me not
to sit still. It tells me I know how
to breathe and act and exercise. It's really
trying to convince me that I can fill +
fix my soul. I don't want to admit that's
what I'm trying to do here. But
it is. This fragile fence I build around
myself in dark times is intended to force
me to feel happy + content.
    The problem is that all this
activity is just an attempt to numb the
painful emptiness. I try to push back the
cloud, make myself forget, or fix it myself.
And in this place of fighting hard +
finding books + pragmatically solving
+ pushing back the cloud, something
murmurs in my heart:
    "Sit with me in the dark."
    But my life is good. I've healed much,
dug deep foundations. This must simply be
chemical, part of a natural predisposition to
depression. If it is natural, why should I
sit in the dark? Why should I engage
the ghosts that haunt, the missing
things + soul-holes that howl around the
sides of consciousness. Life is good. I
want this to be simple. I want to push
through it and call it done for this round.

I was uncomfortable with this invitation to sit in the darkness
and spend some time getting to know the underlying reasons for it.
I feared sitting in my pain because I liked the sense of control that
came when I thought I could manage it all.

By now, I was utterly confident that God was with me and

wouldn't abandon me to the darkness, but I was also convinced the goal was to get out of depression as soon as possible. I feared becoming one who wallows, who chooses to live in self-pity and stays stuck too long.

Still, that gentle invitation wouldn't leave me alone. I began to realize it was an invitation to a season of deep, intentional healing. I knew it would require stillness and opening up my heart in a way I hadn't before, to take a good long look at the roots of pain beneath the decades of depression and suicidal thoughts.

I resisted as long as I could, thinking the fog would lift and I would be okay again. Instead, the clouds grew thicker. Like twilight arrives slowly until all at once it's pitch black and you realize the sky had been losing light for some time, I found myself slowly then all at once overcome by the darkness.[1]

Finally, it clicked. I wasn't going to be able to overcome it on my own. It wasn't circumstantial, simply the result of a too-busy schedule or a stressful season. Sure, stress would make it worse and I'd been learning to live with my limp, but there was more. I needed to dig down, find the root of the darkness, and learn what it meant for me. I needed to accept the invitation to sit in the dark for a while.

When Psalm 46:10 tells us, "Be still, and know that I am God," our tendency is to think of being still and listening to God in prayer. But other translations add more color and depth to our understanding. Instead of just "be still," we're told to cease striving, calm down, and stop fighting. The Hebrew word translated as "be still" can also mean to relax or let go.[2] In the midst of a song of praise about the power of God and his nearness to help his people is this simple reminder to let go and relax.

While this psalm wasn't originally about mental health, it does reveal something important about the character and heart of God. We can let our guards down with him. We don't have to try to hide the darkness (or any struggle or brokenness) or handle it all on our own. He wants to help us navigate a path toward greater wholeness. And sometimes it takes a while. Sometimes, the transformation isn't immediate.

Long ago, the people of God were taken into captivity in a foreign land. After a brutal siege that decimated the people with disease and starvation, those who survived were taken from their homeland.[3] False prophets were promising freedom and deliverance would come soon, but God told them that wasn't the case. "Do not listen to the dreams that they dream," God said, "for it is a lie that they are prophesying to you in my name; I did not send them" (Jeremiah 29:8–9).

Instead, God told them to settle in for the long term, to build houses, plant gardens, and even get married and start families because it was going to be a while. In fact, they would be in Babylon for seventy years. And into that context, God spoke the words that have become so well known: "For I know the plans I have for you, declares the LORD, plans for welfare and not for evil, to give you a future and a hope" (verse 11).

So often, we want to skip straight to the future and hope. We want to move right past the process and cling to the promise. But it doesn't work that way. Sometimes, we have to sit still, let go, and stop fighting. Sometimes, we have to settle in when we feel like we're in exile and learn to thrive where we are. And for those of us with severe depression, that means we might need to settle in and get comfortable in the confusion and uncertainty of the darkness. But that doesn't mean we don't take action when needed; if we're experiencing intense suicidal thoughts and can't stay safe on our own, we need to seek professional help right away. Settling in is just a way of recognizing that we probably won't be packing our bags and leaving exile tomorrow, so we do our best to engage the process where we are.

Up until this point, I had leaned heavily on the church for my healing. I had never spoken to a doctor about the darkness. I hadn't worked with a counselor long term as part of my healing process. Instead, I'd done tons of praying, studying, confessing, trying to change things all the ways I (and my friends and leaders) knew how. I'd "released things to the Lord" and "practiced forgiveness." I'd learned to slow down in ministry, to move at a more sustainable pace.

Even when I was surrounded by an incredible community that loved and accepted me, I still struggled. Those wonderful relationships couldn't heal me on their own. I needed to deal with other factors: my unresolved trauma, lies I believed about myself and about God, and hidden habits that were undermining my progress toward wholeness. Those wounds don't just go away on their own.

It's Not Just Chemical

You may have had a similar experience with trying to heal from mental illness. No matter how you've prayed, read your Bible, and built community, the darkness remains. That doesn't mean there's anything wrong with you. Mental health is much more complicated than that.

Despite the stigma that remains in the church, the wider culture has become fairly familiar with the chemical imbalance theory of mental illness. It's become much more accepted because of pharmaceutical ads—when we see ads explaining that antidepressants can help overcome depression by increasing the serotonin (or other chemicals) in the brain, it makes sense. In many ways, the chemical imbalance theory has helped fight stigma by making mental illness seem as simple and physical as something like diabetes. Unfortunately, it offers an incomplete picture.

Researchers and mental health professionals now know that it's not as simple as a serotonin deficiency. There are many causes for mental illnesses, and it's often a complicated mix of factors that result in one person becoming dangerously depressed and suicidal and another seeming to take life in stride. Genetics, stress, other medical issues, and traumatic experiences can all contribute to depression.[4]

For those who deal with this howling darkness, trauma is a major factor. In fact, one study found that more than 75 percent of patients with chronic depression had experienced significant trauma in childhood. When we hear about trauma, we may think about extreme situations: war, assault, severe abuse, or neglect. But the psychological threshold for trauma can actually be much lower. It's anything that overwhelms our ability to cope, floods us with anxiety and helplessness, and undermines our sense of safety. That doesn't just have to be physical abuse; emotional abuse and neglect have also been found to increase the lifetime risk of depression.[5]

One of the hallmarks of trauma is a deep desire to avoid things that remind us of the overwhelming experiences. It's not fun to dig into those painful experiences; in some cases, it's outright terrifying. So we do the best we can to protect ourselves from reliving the trauma. We might try to deny, minimize, or normalize the events, saying things like "It wasn't that bad. Others have it much worse." We may avoid discussing it altogether, if we can.[6]

For those of us who have some underlying trauma, the last thing we want to do is dig into it. After a lifetime of being fed perfectionism and curated images, the prospect of opening the deepest and most painful wounds of the heart is terrifying. We want to believe we're past the scary, sad, confusing stuff we've experienced. We want to believe it doesn't change how we live today.

But if more than 75 percent of those who deal with the darkness endured overwhelming events in childhood—and that doesn't include trauma experienced as adults—it's no wonder that we need to sit with it and find additional support to find healing. Even if we don't have a lot of big-T trauma (the events we think of as traumatic: war, assault, natural disasters, and so on), most of us still carry some tender, broken pieces we would *really* prefer to keep hidden.

Maybe you hear this invitation to sit in the dark for a while, to partner with God in your healing process, and you immediately think of some things you'd rather God not put a finger on, *thank you very much*. Or maybe nothing major comes to mind, but you know you haven't been able to find wholeness with all the things you've tried up to this point.

———

In my role at the therapeutic home, I kept coming face to face with my own unresolved trauma. So much so that I soon learned I couldn't run any longer. By that point, I had picked up some skills I needed to survive in the dark, and for a while that included fighting like mad to get out of it as soon as possible. But I also discovered that the tools and skills that had gotten me this far wouldn't take me further.

The good news is that there are very learnable skills that move us beyond surviving and into thriving. I wasn't able to learn them on my own. I discovered how badly I needed help, both from God and from mental health professionals. And if you want to move from surviving into thriving, my bet is you'll need some help too. This is especially true if you might have some unresolved trauma to work through, as so many of us do.

I hope you're already working with a team of wise, compassionate professionals. If not, this is your moment to start. Yes, it can be scary. Yes, it might feel like choosing to sit in the dark instead of reaching for the light. But this is where you discover the power of partnering with the Lord in your own healing. This is where you surrender to the gifts God has given us—therapists, doctors, medications, and other treatments—to find restoration you never knew was possible.

You're going to make room to deal with the sources of your depression, anxiety, and suicidal thoughts in the presence of wise professionals and a God who refuses to give up on you. You're about to discover that, even if you have to live with a limp for the rest of your life, it doesn't have to be nearly as difficult or painful as it is now. You're about to discover hope in the dark that you couldn't have imagined.

These may sound like big promises, and I don't blame you if you doubt them. I wouldn't have believed them at the start of my journey. But, my dear friend, if I can do this, so can you. It's hard work that requires good support, and sometimes it fiercely hurts, but it's worth it. It really can get better. This is why that growth mindset we talked about early on is so essential, why it looks so much like the hope that keeps us drawing breath another day. We've got to cling to the belief that we can learn and grow and change even in the midst of our pain.

Listen, I know the expectations of social media–saturated culture make it difficult to let our guards down, even with God. We are supposed to be hardworking hustlers, faithful show-uppers, joyful believers who talk about how well we're blessed. In work, in life, in church—in so many places, for so many people, we feel this pressure to push down the fears and doubts and aches. So we build walls to keep others out, including God. We've become accustomed to painting bright colors over our darkness, trying to hide it even, if possible, from ourselves.

True healing, though, doesn't come from resistance. Vulnerability with God, with loved ones, and with good professionals can feel like choosing to sit in a pitch-black room instead of reaching for the light—and how can we choose to sit when everything in us says to run and move and make things happen?

But if we accept the invitation, we can find the power of partnering with the Lord in our own healing. We choose to make room to deal with possible sources of depression and suicidal thoughts. And the surprising thing is that taking the time to sit with the darkness can actually empower us to participate in the work of healing God wants to do in us.

Twelve

When Provision Comes in a Pill

My hands shook as I stared at the phone, sick with dread. Hiding in my car after a long shift at the residential facility, I was frightened and embarrassed to make this call. But I was terrified of what would happen if I didn't.

The dark thoughts were becoming vicious, graphic, and much more intrusive. Dozens of times each day, my mind was filled with images of self-directed violence, and none of my coping skills could get them to stop. It's a strange thing to explain thoughts of self-harm and suicide to those who haven't dealt with them. It wasn't something I *wanted* to do, and yet there's this incredibly powerful urge, nearly a compulsion, to the thoughts.

That weekend, they'd reached a new intensity. I was sitting in the office at the residential facility, listening to my coworkers chat about the day. I'd kicked off my shoes and propped my feet on a bench. Suddenly, all I could think about was putting my foot into the paper shredder. Even after dealing with graphic and frightening thoughts for most of my life, I was horrified. That's when I knew I needed help.

Monday morning, right after my shift, I sat in my car and tried to find help. I didn't know who to call; I was new to Nashville and hadn't seen a doctor yet. So I just started scrolling through names of providers online, dialing with my trembling fingers and praying something would work out.

Office after office, I discovered it would take weeks for me to get in. I tried psychiatrists and general practitioners, but no luck. Finally, I called a large health system in the area. Once again, the scheduler told me it would be weeks until there was an opening. I broke down.

My voice was small and shook through my tears. "I don't know if I'm going to be okay that long," I said. The truth was that I already wasn't okay. I just didn't know if I could continue to keep myself safe.

The scheduler's voice softened. "Hang on for me, honey. Let me see what I can do." I waited on hold, trying to breathe deeply and stop sniffling. The scheduler returned and said I could see a doctor in just a few days but it would be a general practitioner since the psychiatrists were booked up. I sighed with relief. She made me promise her that I would go to the emergency room if I needed to. I said I would and ended the call.

———

The doctor was kind, patient, and obviously cared very much. She listened to my story, my struggles and fears, my concerns about side effects, then asked questions about my symptoms and thoughts about hurting myself. I didn't hold anything back; I just wanted to get better. She took all those factors into account, suggested a medication to try, and told me what to expect when I started taking it. Before I left, she talked to me about warning signs, encouraged me to start therapy, talked about when to go to the emergency room for suicidal thoughts, and made sure I knew how to contact her in case I needed anything.

I remember finding my way back to my car in the parking garage, feeling a tiny sliver of hope in my chest. I was still aching, overwhelmed, and filled with anxiety that felt like constant terror. But the thing that stuck out most about that day was the kindness and compassion of the doctor.

I was lucky; while it can take several weeks for antidepressants to take effect, I started noticing some changes within days. I felt a little funny at first, as if I were wearing glasses and the prescription was a bit off, and much more tired than normal. I emailed my doctor, who suggested I change the time of day I took the meds, and the fatigue started to dissipate. Before long, the clouds began to lift as well.

Why didn't I do this sooner?

Taking medication for depression is difficult to write about. People have big opinions about it, and those opinions aren't always based on sound science. But even experts disagree on how and when they should be used. Some people think meds should be frontline defense for anybody dealing with mental health issues. Others think they should be used as a last resort. Many fall somewhere in between.

Of course, as a Christian, I dealt with the stigma that told me taking medication meant I lacked faith for God to heal me and I lacked the strength of character to make life changes that would lead to wellness.

People talk about exercise and eating well, but sometimes I couldn't get off the couch. Sometimes I was so nauseous with anxiety that I couldn't eat at all. So, for many years, I bought the lie that if I couldn't get better without medication, something was really wrong with me. Finally, when the searing shadows became too much, I gave in and made the call.

I'm so glad I did.

God's Not Upset

We need to settle something: seeking medical care for mental illness—or any illness—is not a lack of faith or a rejection of God's provision. Good doctors, scientific research, and advances in health technologies often *are* his provision.

There's a dangerous double standard when it comes to mental health care. We don't say people lack faith when they depend on lifesaving medications like insulin for diabetes, an inhaler for asthma, or an EpiPen for extreme allergic reactions. And we certainly don't shame them for talking to doctors about their illnesses. We are grateful that our family members receive good medical treatment and that we live in a world where things that used to kill many people are now very manageable.

But perhaps because we still don't think of mental illnesses as *real* diseases, many believers don't see it the same way. We are more hesitant to thank God for the lifesaving medications that prevent tragic deaths by suicide. We suddenly develop amnesia, forgetting how often the Lord works through the knowledge and wisdom he's given to humankind.

The good news is that we can look to Scripture to be reminded. There are plenty of references to doctors and medicine in the Bible. We know that Luke, author of one of the gospels and the book of Acts, was known as "the beloved physician"; as a doctor, he was a valued and beloved part of the early church. Paul told Timothy to use a little wine as medicine for his stomach. Joseph commanded the doctors in Egypt to take care of his father's body. Jeremiah used a lack of medicine to heal as a metaphor for irreparable damage done to his people (Colossians 4:14; 1 Timothy 5:23; Genesis 50:2; Jeremiah 8:22; 30:13; 46:11).

Even Jesus talked about doctors, using them to illustrate his mission. "Healthy people don't need a doctor," he said, but "sick people do. I have come to call not those who think they are righteous, but those who know they are sinners and need to repent." Another time, he referenced a common phrase people used in his time: "Physician, heal yourself" (Luke 5:31–32, NLT; Luke 4:23). Jesus was speaking specifically about whether or not he would perform miracles in his hometown, so this was more about a figure of speech than literal doctors.

But what stands out to me is that, in all these verses, plus many more that casually mention doctors and medicines, we don't get a sense that God condemns people for seeking medical help. God's not disappointed in you for getting the help you need.

What to Know About Working with a Doctor

When I finally saw a doctor about my lifelong depression, I was afraid. I remembered those old messages I'd heard about taking meds being a sign of a lack of faith, and part of me was disappointed in myself for needing them. But I've since learned that medication can be an important part of a holistic treatment plan. And for some of us who wrestle with the darkness, they can be the very provision of God that we've been praying for.

Stigma in and out of the church means that mental illnesses are seriously undertreated in our culture. The National Institute of Mental Health estimated that 35 percent of adults who experienced a major depressive episode in 2017 didn't receive any treatment; that number jumped to more than 60 percent for adolescents (tweens and teens).[1] At the same time, suicide rates are increasing dramatically, and more than half of those who die by suicide don't have a diagnosed mental illness.[2]

Stigma and undertreatment of mental illnesses are leading to preventable suicides every single day: they prevent us from seeking help, make us less likely to continue with lifesaving treatments, and make us feel more isolated. When stigma says it's not okay to talk about our pain, that we will be seen as "crazy," and that others will reject us, we're far less likely to open up and find the support that could save our lives.[3] We've got to change those statistics. This is why everybody who struggles with his mental health needs to work with well-equipped health care providers.

It's a good idea to start by reaching out to your primary care physician and talking about what you're experiencing. More than likely, your doctor will want to rule out any other conditions that could cause depressive symptoms. Thyroid problems, head injuries, strokes, seizures, Lyme disease, and many others have been linked to symptoms of depression, as have several vitamin and mineral deficiencies. Other medications can also cause symptoms, so it's important to get a good checkup and talk to your doctor about all symptoms you're experiencing.[4]

If everything else checks out medically, you can work with your doctor to find a good treatment plan that works for you. Treatment doesn't necessarily mean medication; it just means working with a trained health care provider to come up with a plan to move toward wholeness. There are plenty of evidence-based options available, and a good doctor can help you find something that works for you. Research has shown that some supplements can be helpful in depression.[5] Many health care providers are familiar with other complementary treatments that might be helpful; things like light therapy, exercise, and even acupuncture have been shown to positively impact depression.[6] There is even emerging research that suggests dietary changes can reduce symptoms of depression.[7]

But it's also okay to decide that you want to try medication. Your general practitioner may be willing to write a prescription for you, or she might refer you to a psychiatrist, especially if the first medication you try doesn't work for you. Psychiatrists are trained and experienced in the finer details of medications, side effects, and more severe mental health issues your primary care provider may misdiagnose, and it's great to have one on your mental health team. In fact, it's ideal to start working with a psychiatrist as soon as you're able, so you can benefit from the wisdom of a specialist intimately acquainted with treating your condition, especially for long-term care.

Antidepressants made a huge difference for me, and they do for the majority of people who take them. Though it seems strange, we don't entirely understand how they work. As I've mentioned, scientists now know that the chemical imbalance theory of depression is incomplete. There's increasing evidence that depression is linked to inflammation in the body; antidepressants have been shown to decrease inflammation.[8] They also seem to help increase neuroplasticity (the brain's ability to change itself), alter the way neurotransmitters work in the brain, and increase its ability to learn through things like therapy.[9]

While the intricate workings of our brains and bodies still hold plenty of mystery, we do know that medication can be a helpful component of treatment. Most people who take antidepressants see a significant improvement in symptoms within two months.[10] They can also prevent relapses when continued after depression goes into remission.[11] While mild to moderate depression can often be treated with therapy alone, most severe depression improves best when treated with a combination of therapy and medication.[12]

Of course, antidepressants aren't perfect. Medications tend to be more effective for severe depression than mild cases.[13] About 60 to 70 percent of patients respond to antidepressants; sometimes, you need to try a few different options before one (or a combination of meds) works. For me, after about a year on my first medication, my doctor and I decided to add a second to help me feel even better. People with treatment-resistant depression often need to try other treatment options or add multiple medications.[14]

Like most medications, antidepressants do come with side effects, but these can sometimes be mitigated by trying a different medication or adjusting the dose. Depending on the severity of your depression and the side effects you experience, you might determine that the side effects aren't worth the possible benefit. That's okay, but that should be a well-informed decision made with a good doctor.

You might have heard about black box warnings or that antidepressants increase suicide risk in teens and young adults. There's a lot of concern about antidepressant use in teens and adolescents due to a black box warning the FDA placed on these medications. Unfortunately, this has led to some confusion and more stigma around medication. The warning came after a study found that teens taking

SSRIs may be 2 percent more likely to experience suicidal thoughts or attempts than those receiving a placebo (though none of the teens actually died by suicide). Obviously, this is concerning and has led many parents to second-guess whether medication is a safe choice for their children. However, untreated depression is a much greater risk factor for suicide than SSRI usage. That's why the FDA warning was intended to make sure teens are closely monitored for suicidal thoughts, not to scare people away from meds.[15] If your kid takes antidepressants, be sure to check in with him, letting him know that if those thoughts come up, your doctor might be able to find another option to better treat him. Of course, if he (or anyone) has new or increasing thoughts of suicide or death, call a doctor immediately for advice.

Finally, it's important to know that it can be difficult to stop taking antidepressants. About 20 percent of patients develop unpleasant symptoms when they abruptly reduce the dose or stop taking them altogether. These symptoms vary based on the medication, are usually mild (but not always), and can often be prevented or reduced with a slow taper.[16]

When Micah and I started thinking about having kids, I met with my doctor to discuss what we should do about my antidepressants. We weighed the factors specific to my situation: one of my medications carried a very small risk of harm to an unborn baby, but we knew it worked well for me; I hadn't experienced a depressive episode in well over a year; and there are other medications that are considered safer in pregnancy. Because I was in such a stable, healthy place, my doctor and I decided together that I was ready to try coming off my antidepressants, knowing I could always start taking them again if necessary. We also decided that I could continue to take my low-dose anxiety medication on an as-needed basis.

Because I had experienced dizziness and nausea if I'd accidentally missed a dose, I tapered off my antidepressants very slowly. It wound up taking about nine months; toward the end, I had quite a bit of vertigo, so the pace slowed to a crawl. It wasn't fun, but the process was worth it for me. And if the day comes that I need those meds again, I will welcome them with gratitude for the provision of science that helps me be well. In the meantime, I will focus on other ways to control my depression, being ruthless with self-care.

Medication isn't right for everyone—this is true. I've been shocked how often this tidbit is highly emphasized in Christian books and resources that talk about mental health. But the part that doesn't show up in many of those books is that, to those of us dealing with severe mental illness, *any* chance of getting better is worth exploring. I finally realized that an imperfect chance of feeling better was absolutely better than continuing to live in such anguish.

For me, it was a lifesaver in one of the most difficult seasons of my life. I wish I had spoken with a doctor about my depression years earlier instead of suffering in silence. When I finally did start medication, I was shocked at how much better I felt. But I also quickly discovered it didn't take away my problems. Instead, it brought the bottom up, made it so the lows weren't so low, and stabilized me enough that I could do the hard work I needed to do in my life.

I still needed to show up to therapy, learn to take care of myself, and make some significant lifestyle changes (all of which we will discuss in the next few chapters). But for me, I didn't have the energy, mental capacity, or overall health to tackle any of those issues until I started taking antidepressants. I love what Dr. Curt Thompson says about this in a story about a patient taking medication long term:

> This pharmacologic intervention supports the ongoing work she is doing to work out her salvation and become the woman God longs for her to be. I often remind her, as I remind all my patients, that it is never my goal for them to be on or off medication. My goal is for them to be well.[17]

For many of us, medications support us as we find the stability required to start healing. This is what is missing from much of the discussion around antidepressants: even if they don't fix your problems, they might be just what you need so that you can get out of bed, go to work, go to therapy, and go on a walk. If you're hesitant to talk to your doctor about meds, it can help to know they can be a temporary part of your path to wellness. They might be what you need to start eating healthier, deal with the trauma, start practicing mindfulness, set boundaries, make a job change—in short, for some people, medication can be an important part of getting to a place where medication isn't needed.

But, just as Dr. Thompson said, the goal isn't to either be on or off meds. The goal is to be healthy, and for many people, that means faithfully taking a medication. There's nothing wrong with you, my friend, if caring for your mental health requires you to swallow those little pills every single day. And if that's you, I rejoice with you that there's something to help you live well despite your diagnosis.

And for some of us, it becomes a lifeline, a miracle, the very provision of God. It can be part of the healing we've longed for.

Thirteen

Good Therapy and Doing the Work

I was 90 percent sure I was going to vomit as I sat in the waiting room. After a few too many bad fits and hurtful experiences with therapy, I was so scared to try again. But this time around, I was committed to doing whatever it took to get better. That meant I had to stay put, no matter how much I wanted to bolt for the door.

I'd gotten her name and number from Shelly, a respected friend who worked in the mental health field, loved people, and reminded me of Jesus. I knew Shelly well enough to know she wouldn't give me a terrible recommendation. But I also knew by now that sometimes it's not the right fit, so I just committed internally to three sessions. Surely by the third session, I would have an idea of whether it was a good fit or not.

I don't remember what made me decide to keep going, but there were so many reasons to have hope. She offered a free consultation so we could both determine if it was a good fit. She was patient and gentle, leaving me space to think and gather the courage to speak, not needing to fill the tense silence. And she was fully present with me in a way I can't explain, other than to say I could tell she brought her whole self to the counseling room.

She explained her style and theory, told me about some different tools we could try, and let me lead. She knew when to back off and when to gently push. She noticed when I started to get anxious and more than once suggested we take a break, talk about something fun, or step outside for some fresh air.

She asked good questions, listened deeper than anyone I've ever met, and reflected my unconscious beliefs back to me so I could see them for what they were. We didn't just talk about my current struggles with depression and thoughts of suicide or self-harm; we looked at long-hidden threads woven throughout my life, pulled on them until we found the end, and learned where the darkness came from together. We used special techniques to process unresolved trauma. The nightmares came less often, and the near-daily panic attacks slowed their furious pace. I was getting better.

After years of painful experiences with therapy and not finding the right fit, I finally had a wonderful counselor. She helped me work through the wrong beliefs and thought patterns, trauma, and unhealthy habits. It wasn't easy; showing up to counseling every week can be hard, draining work. There were times I wanted to quit because of the difficult memories and emotions that came up in sessions. But as Jenna walked with me toward wholeness, I was able to experience healing that I had never imagined.

Then she went on sabbatical, and I needed to find a new therapist.

I don't think people talk often enough about how tough it can be to change counselors. I was sad and disappointed at first. I didn't want to go through the whole process of finding someone new, figuring out if it was a good fit, and telling my story all over again. Honestly, I grieved a little bit after my time with Jenna ended.

Still, after a few weeks, I found someone new to work with. And it's been so good for me. Megan, my current therapist, has a very different personality and style than Jenna. It took a little longer for me to fall into a rhythm and to feel comfortable with her, but that has taught me so much.

I've learned to advocate better for myself and to build a healthy relationship. I had to learn to ask for what I needed in ways I wasn't used to. At one point, I felt like I wasn't making much progress and suspected I would benefit from a slight adjustment in the format of our sessions. I was so nervous to tell my counselor something wasn't working for me; I half expected her to tell me it was my fault, as another counselor had years earlier. But when I asked, Megan responded with delight that I had talked to her about it. And I'm so glad I did. Not only did I move past the plateau and start growing more, I learned that relationships—both personal and professional—could benefit from me having the courage to be honest and ask for what I needed.

The lessons and breakthroughs that happen in therapy can help *anyone* have a happier, healthier life and relationships. But it's especially important for those of us who deal with the darkness to partner with someone to walk toward wholeness.

For most of us, trying to treat the symptoms of depression is not enough. It's not enough to just look at what we're currently dealing with—the brain fog and sadness, the apathy and exhaustion—and try to treat it with medication and lifestyle changes. If we're to ever find wholeness, we're going to need to dig deeper into the foundations of our illnesses. In other words, we can't get well if we won't deal with our trauma, the lies we believe, the bitterness or pain we may hold, and our unhealthy coping mechanisms.

A Sacred Invitation

Before I started working in the mental health field and seeing good therapists, I didn't understand just how much the beautiful beating heart of God is wholly, fully for restoration. Sure, I saw it in Scripture, in that best-beloved psalm that we whisper in the valley of the shadow, scarcely daring to hope it could be true: "He restores my soul" (Psalm 23:3). But it wasn't until I watched those young women walking the hard road of healing—and walked my own in counseling—that I began to see the way the Lord offers the sacred invitation to participate in his work of restoration.

In all my years of praying for God to wave his magic wand and fix me, I missed that sacred invitation. I missed the way even miracles require the recipient to take a step on faltering, unsteady legs. I thought miracles happened in a single moment, that there was always a line of demarcation between "before" and "after." But as I watched those young women take stumbling steps toward greater wholeness—showing up at the residential counseling home, faithfully attending therapy sessions, and imperfectly implementing what they learned—I saw them transformed in marvelous ways. And when I gained the courage to accept that sacred invitation, countless stories from the Bible held new meaning for me.

Just as God made a miraculous way of escape for the Israelites from Egypt, so he has made a way for us. But Israel had to obey, pack their things, and start walking. They had to participate (Exodus 12–14). Then, when it was time for Israel to enter the promised land, the priests had to step into the river, carrying the ark, before the waters would dry up and the whole nation could cross over (Joshua 3). Nehemiah had to participate by speaking to the king and rebuilding the wall before Jerusalem could be restored (Nehemiah 1–2). When Naaman wanted to be healed from leprosy, it didn't happen right away; he had to wash seven times in the Jordan River (2 Kings 5:1–14). When the angel came to rescue Peter from prison, Peter had to get up, get dressed, and follow, even though he wasn't sure if he could believe his eyes (Acts 12:7–9).

Over and over in Scripture, God shows how he wants us to join him in his work of restoration in the world—and our lives. He is gentle and kind; he won't force us to participate. But so often, he invites us to take a step of faith, to cooperate with the good work he wants to do in our lives and in the world around us. And for those of us who battle mental illness, that step of faith may look like setting an appointment, showing up consistently, and joining him in the good work of restoration in our own lives.

How to Do the Work

There are no real shortcuts in moving toward wholeness, just hard work empowered by the Holy Spirit.[1] The same is true of working with a counselor or therapist. I know what it feels like to work so hard to get better. The reality is that when we think we're working so hard to change, we're often spinning our wheels, reinforcing the patterns and states that keep us locked in our anguish.[2] But working with a good therapist can open up new ways of working through those difficult patterns.

When we're in the process, progress seems slow. It's easy to think that when God doesn't heal instantly, we're not experiencing miracles. But working with a compassionate, well-equipped therapist to move toward greater wholeness requires faith. And engaging that process in faith and faithfully often leads to results that seem pretty miraculous.

Neuroscientists are discovering that counseling can actually change circuits in our brains. It increases focus, reduces anxiety and depression, and helps us reconnect with joy.[3] Different types of therapy can change the levels of activity in different parts of the brain that are linked to anxiety, worry, the ability to feel pleasure, optimism, and behaviors that contribute to depression.

Therapy works on different circuits and structures in the brain than medication does; for example, talk therapy can change activity in the limbic system (which is responsible for our emotions, among other things). That's one of the reasons why, for those severely depressed, a combination of medication and therapy can be way more effective than just one or the other. Plus, therapists can also act as coaches, empowering us and providing more tools we can use to get better.[4]

All of this means that sitting on a couch in a counselor's office is about way more than just talking. I've made a great deal of progress through therapy and have found a level of wholeness that is, frankly, an answer to many prayers I've prayed. While I was praying for God to restore my soul, expecting it to happen in an instant, I didn't know he was inviting me to join in that process. Therapy helps us tap into the God-given capability of our brains and bodies to heal.

So how do we make therapy work for us?

Remember, the most important factor is having a good relationship with your therapist.[5] One of the most powerful things we can experience is being seen, known, and unjudged. The counseling room becomes a safe space with a safe person who can reflect back our thoughts, feelings, and experiences to help us make meaning of them. What is wounded in relationship must also be healed in relationship,[6] and we have the opportunity to do that in our work with compassionate, well-trained therapists.

Beyond the relational aspects of therapy, there are different techniques (sometimes called modalities) that might work better for people with certain diagnoses or more severe mental illness. For example, a mindfulness-based approach can be especially helpful if you've had multiple depressive episodes.[7] Cognitive behavioral therapy (CBT) is a well-known modality that focuses on the negative thought patterns we often experience with depression. It's also very well researched, so there's lots of evidence that it can be really helpful.[8]

One approach that can be especially helpful for those of us with severe depression, multiple mental health diagnoses, or intense suicidal thoughts is called dialectical behavioral therapy. DBT is a multilayered approach that was originally developed to treat borderline personality disorder, but research has shown it can help reduce suicide attempts and self-harm. It incorporates mindfulness, acceptance, and problem-solving skills to help people cope with the painful emotions and experiences that make suicide and self-harm seem like the only options.[9] It's a specialized type of therapy, so if this sounds right for you, you'll need to find somebody trained in it.

Many therapists are trained in multiple types of therapy and experiment to combine what's helpful for you as an individual. This is another reason your relationship with your counselor is so important; when it's a trusting partnership working toward a mutual goal, it's much easier to explore what works for you.

My experience as a client, working in a residential mental health facility, and talking with others who struggle in the dark has made me a major advocate for trauma-informed therapy, simply because trauma is so exceedingly common. While we might not think of ourselves as trauma survivors, most of us would benefit from the special tools in this type of therapy. Remember, more than three-fourths of people with depression have a significant history of traumatic experiences. And, even if we don't think of our experiences as particularly harrowing, our implicit memory records information below the conscious level in our brains that impacts how we respond and act. Any event that overwhelms our ability to cope can be traumatic, leaving unseen bits and pieces of pain buried in implicit memory and hindering our ability to move forward in healing.

Trauma-informed therapists understand how overwhelming experiences change our brains and bodies.[10] They pay special attention to making sure we feel safe and empowered, and they're usually trained in special techniques to help us reprocess those difficult bits of traumatic memory. Techniques like EMDR, or eye movement desensitization and reprocessing, and brainspotting are brain-based therapies designed to help process and heal unresolved trauma. Looking for a therapist trained in EMDR and similar modalities or who specializes in trauma can make a world of difference in helping you get unstuck, just as it did for me.

One common thread in all the counselors I saw who weren't a right fit for me (aside from the one who wasn't actually licensed) was that they weren't trauma-informed. The difference was stark when I started working with Jenna, who happened to be both brilliant at wading through the aftermath of trauma, and a Christian. As a note, it can be a great blessing to work with Christian counselors. But it's much more important that they're trained, licensed, and well equipped than that they believe the same things about God as you. (If you need help finding a good therapist, please see chapter 5 for tips on finding the right fit.)

What to Know About Working with a Therapist

You've found a counselor and you've made an appointment. Great! Now what? This may sound silly, but the first thing is to commit to showing up. Remember, it can take a few sessions to feel comfortable with a new therapist, so committing to three sessions (barring any red flags, as discussed in chapter 5) gives you time to decide if it's a good fit. By then, you should start to feel safer opening up with your therapist if it's a good fit.

Next, know that therapy will get easier as you gain experience. You may feel uncomfortable and it will probably be awkward at first; you might not be sure what to say or how to relate to your counselor. That's totally normal, considering this is a different type of relationship than any other in your life. Show up every week, even if it's awkward. Consistent therapy will lead to the best outcomes and help you make progress more quickly. This is especially true if you're in a severe depressive episode or changing medications (which should always be done with medical supervision).

Sessions may flow differently based on your therapist's style. She may start with a question like "What are you bringing in today?" or "What would you like to talk about today?" My current counselor often starts sessions with a minute or two of small talk, then asks me to check in with myself to share what I'm thinking and feeling.

There may be a lot of silence as she waits for you to process and speak. I expected a lot more advice at first, so I initially found the patient stillness unnerving. Over time, I learned I really need that space to think, breathe, and listen to what's going on inside me. I've grown to love it and have even asked for it when I felt like we were filling too much space.

Your therapist should practice very good, professional boundaries and keep the focus of the session on you. At times, it may seem strange that she knows so much about you and you know so little about her personal life, but it's okay. She's there to help you, so she probably won't share too much.

She may occasionally offer a story from her own life when it's clearly relevant and benefits you. My current therapist recently shared an example from her life to help me navigate a conflict. Before she offered it, she said, "I have a story from my own life that may be helpful if you're open to hearing it." I gave permission before she proceeded.

You shouldn't feel the need to support your counselor in any way. Some of us naturally fall into the role of a caretaker, so it can be tough to resist, but your therapist should never make you feel like you're her confidant or there to care for her.

Your therapist should never name another client's name. This should go without saying, but licensed mental health professionals are bound by privacy laws, just like doctors. You can be sure that if a counselor mentions another client by name to you, she'll mention you by name to someone else.

An important part of doing the work in therapy is realizing that you have a ton of control in the process. Your therapist is not the boss of you and is not 100 percent in charge of the sessions. You decide what to share and when; you get to express preferences and ask for what you need. If something's not working for you, you can ask for reasonable adjustments. If it's not something that works for your therapist, she should discuss it with you and you should find a compromise or realize she's not a good fit.

A good counselor will help you discover what's most helpful for you. She may have suggestions of coping skills, homework assignments, books to read, or activities to try, but this is not an authority figure for you to blindly submit to. Nor should the interaction feel overly familiar, such as the relationship you have with a best friend. Instead, it's helpful to view mental health professionals as partners on your journey to healing. Again, professional boundaries are a key part of the therapeutic relationship. Sometimes they're tough to navigate, especially if we've experienced abandonment, neglect, or other deep wounds. But these boundaries help us grow and become healthier, so they're absolutely essential

Try not to worry about what your therapist will think about the things you say. More than likely, she's heard something similar before. When I started working with Jenna, I made a commitment to bring complete honesty to my sessions. There were definitely thoughts and feelings I didn't want to bring up, but I promised myself I would say the things I was afraid to. I realized that, even when I was hesitant to say whatever came to mind, she could help me sift through all my thoughts, feelings, and experiences to find what would be most helpful to focus on.

I've carried that practice into my current counseling relationship, and I'm convinced it helps us work through hard stuff much more easily because we're facing it head-on together. At times, I say things like "I feel afraid/ashamed/embarrassed to say this, but . . ." or "When you said that, I noticed I thought or felt . . ." I'll speak up if something she says doesn't resonate with me because I've learned that it doesn't help us make progress if I stay silent.

I always mention any thoughts of suicide or self-harm that come up. I know we can fear what will happen if we're honest about what's really going on inside. But talking about scary stuff, even suicide, can take a lot of the power of shame out of it.

You may have heard stories of people mentioning thoughts of suicide to a therapist and then winding up in a hospital. A good mental health professional should be able to talk through your struggles and help you evaluate your suicide risk. A lot of times, that means having productive conversations about how to keep yourself safe and cope when those intrusive thoughts do show up.

But if you're really not able to stay safe (such as if you have a plan or access to lethal means to end your life), the safest place might be a hospital for a little while. *That's absolutely okay.* Having a good therapist on your team means having somebody who can help you navigate the options you have as you learn to live well despite the darkness. You don't have to figure it out on your own.

One final tip: if possible, schedule your counseling appointments during a time when you won't need to be "on" so much immediately afterward. You'll often want a little breathing room after appointments that may be tough or leave you feeling emotionally vulnerable. In difficult seasons, I choose not to make any firm commitments (like going to dinner with friends) for after counseling because I know I might want to cancel. Instead, prioritize some soothing self-care time. This makes it easier to integrate the growth from your sessions into your everyday life.

———

I've come a long way from that anxious day when I thought I was going to throw up all over the waiting room. Now I've been going to therapy faithfully for four years, only missing a session if I was ill or out of town.

When I started going to counseling regularly, I'd been stuck for so long that I didn't know if I could ever overcome so many of the things that kept me bound to the deepest darkness. Therapy has taught me to change toxic beliefs and thought patterns, work through unresolved trauma, and find healthier coping mechanisms for my worst days.

I want that for you too. I want you to get to the point that your darkest memories don't haunt you anymore, that the most painful moments of your life don't hold quite the same power. I want you to experience the healing power that God has embedded in relationships and the tools given to mental health professionals.

If counseling hasn't worked for you in the past, that's okay. It took me five attempts before I found the right therapist for me. My hope is that the information I've shared in this chapter will help you find a great fit sooner and see your counselor as a partner who walks with you on the path to healing.

As you do, I pray you will discover the same thing I did: that the very natural means God has provided for our mental health can be the miracles we've been looking for all along.

Fourteen

Beating Back the Darkness

It's okay. I shut the heavy door behind me, listening for the click of the lock that meant nobody could come in and see me fall apart. Something was trying to claw its way out of my chest, and I couldn't stop shuddering. I pressed my back to the door and slid down it, crumpling into a fetal curl on the floor.

You're doing the best you can. That's more than enough. I squeezed myself in a tight embrace on the meds room floor, whispered the words into the cavern in my chest, speaking peace into the storm. I wasn't used to this yet. It felt wrong, selfish, and like I was letting myself off the hook when I should have been trying harder.

But my skin burned with shame as images of self-harm bubbled up in my mind. So I kept at it, picturing the faces of young women I worked with, imagining the kind words that would have been easy to extend to them.

I'm not disappointed in you. I know this hurts and it's so hard, but it's going to get better. Dark days don't last forever. Keep going. You're doing a good job.

I was often assigned to that meds room in my work at the residential facility for young women with mental health issues. Morning, noon, and night, they filed in one at a time while I carefully dispensed medications from the locked cabinet, made sure they swallowed their pills, and logged each dose.

Those few minutes alone with each girl gave me a chance to connect deeper. The girls shared their struggles and stories. I saw their shame, their fear, their anguish. Often, I was the first to see their self-inflicted wounds, the one to clean and care for them when they needed first aid and to hear they weren't terrible humans.

I saw them at their lowest, most vulnerable moments. Still, it was so easy to see all the good. They were full of strength and courage, beauty and wisdom and willingness to learn, even when it was all buried under so much pain. It was obvious that, underneath the unhealthy coping skills, they were fighting for progress. I *knew* their stories weren't over, that they were writing new chapters on healing and wholeness even as they struggled and "messed up." I was so proud of them.

It was so easy to speak life and hope and encouragement to them, to call out their strengths, to remind them that they weren't bad people for struggling and needing help.

But it had never been so easy to speak kindly to myself.

I was in the midst of one of the deepest depressive episodes of my life. I was finally working with a great therapist; I'd become genuinely secure in the love of God and had grown in a sense of self-worth as his child. But that familiar ache exposed harsh beliefs that had been deeply buried. They bubbled to the surface as brutal thoughts: *Why are you so lazy? What's wrong with you? Pull yourself together. This is ridiculous; you just want attention.* And they felt completely justified, even right. *After all, if I'm not hard on myself, who will be? How will I ever get anything done? How will I ever do anything right?*

In therapy, I learned we often develop those beliefs and that sort of internal dialogue to keep ourselves in line and prevent others from being able to punish us. My therapist reminded me that I don't need those beliefs anymore and gently challenged me to see it in a different way.

So I started talking to myself as I talked to those I cared about: my best friend, my sister, the residents at work, my young nieces. It was awkward and uncomfortable, like putting your shoes on the wrong feet.

But it got easier. And my heart slowly softened toward myself. The heaviness began to lighten.

6/5/16

Hope sounds like words I don't feel for myself, piped up from some hard-dug reservoir deep inside. A resident was panicking + came for help. There were many words and tears + prayers, but somewhere in there, I told truth I don't feel for me:

You are lovely. And we see so many beautiful things in you. And sometimes, it doesn't seem possible + the fight is too hard. But it's going to be okay. You aren't stuck here forever. A year from now, you'll look back + wonder how you could ever be so free. You'll be amazed because you didn't know life could feel like that.

And I thought how those words are true for me. My life is already more beautiful than I had hoped, and I'm learning self-care + grace + love. And I know how to sit in the dark now, to still hear your voice of love speaking there.

And it is going to be okay.

This may be the chapter I'm most excited to write because this is where I truly started to thrive. I know that may sound audacious and unreachable, as though thriving isn't for us who wrestle with severe depression. But as I learned to take ownership of my mental health, to care well for myself, and to refuse to live by the old rules that mental illness had taught me, I slowly discovered that life can be good, even in the darkness.

It's inevitable: If you spend much time under the cloud of depression, you get so used to it that you believe its lies. You accept the ugly accusations and cruel self-judgment. Even when you're not fighting off thoughts of self-harm or suicide, there's this harsh soundtrack playing that says you're a worthless failure, nobody can love or want you, life will always be this way, or some other hideous thing we wouldn't say to another person. It may sound a little different for you, but my bet is you know exactly what I'm talking about.

Over time, those lies warp into unspoken rules we live by: *Don't hope. Don't let your guard down; something bad is right around the corner. Don't try (you know you're just going to fail, anyway). Be strict with yourself because that's the only way you'll ever get anything done.*

But learning to thrive despite mental illness requires fighting back against the grim thoughts. We must learn to beat back the darkness.

This is the rubber-meets-the-road, day-by-day process that moved me from death to life, clinging to the hand of God and the support of mental health professionals. This is how I learned to breathe despite the heaviness in my chest, to find joy in the midst of the sadness, and to fight like mad to get better.

I had to learn to disrupt the thought patterns and beliefs that kept me in the deepest pits of depression by doing the opposite of what seemed natural.

When I wanted to belittle myself, I spoke kindly and reminded myself of my belovedness. When I was caught in spiraling anxiety, I wrote lists recounting God's faithfulness in my life and read through lists of my favorite hope-filled Scriptures. And when fear and stigma told me to keep silent about thoughts of suicide and self-harm, I reached out to safe, supportive friends for accountability.

I settled something important in my heart: thoughts of suicide, of worthlessness, and of hurting myself aren't my own true thoughts. They are a symptom of a terrible disease. I had to come to grips with

10/27/19

You are the Beloved

When I sleep	I am the Beloved
When I rise	I am the Beloved
When I am depressed	I am the Beloved
When I'm angry	I am the Beloved

When I fail, I am the Beloved
When I fall, I am the Beloved
When I'm selfish, I am the Beloved.
When I'm grateful, I am the Beloved
When I'm anxious, I am the Beloved
When I lose touch of reality I am the Beloved
When I forget what you sound like,
        I am the Beloved.
When I try to hold the pieces together,
        I am the Beloved.
When I try to do it in my own strength,
        I am the Beloved
and when it all falls apart,
  when I have nothing to offer,
  when I'm naked and ashamed
  and unable to offer a thing to you,

the fact that, even on my worst days and in the midst of suicidal thoughts, I don't really *want* to die. The disease is *telling me* I want to die. That may seem like a subtle difference on paper, but when I began to live from that mindset, everything changed for me.

And I've seen it work for others, for residents I worked with, for friends, and even for readers of my blog. Because it's a game changer to notice these grim, disturbing thoughts and know they're just nasty symptoms of a brutal illness. It makes a world of difference to be able to say something like "I'm having thoughts of self-harm" instead of believing them and thinking, in your heart of hearts, that you *actually* want to stop living.

None of us really wants that; we just want to stop hurting so much. For some believers, this may manifest as a desire to "go be with Jesus." While we relate to Paul's desire "to depart and be with Christ" (Philippians 1:23), that usually comes from a place of longing for our suffering to end. In reality, we don't want to miss out on the millions of beautiful moments that make up a life: laughter and smiles, the warmth of sunlight and love, a future with purpose, hope, and people we care about. We just don't want our lives to be controlled by unending darkness and pain.

The good news is that we don't have to miss out on any of that. We can truly shake off the tyrannical control of mental illness, even if it doesn't fully disappear, as we learn to beat back the darkness.

In my life, I've found two main areas to focus on. In this chapter, we'll look at beating back the darkness internally. We'll talk about ways to disrupt the thought patterns and lies that are symptoms of mental illness through simple practices that make our minds a much nicer place to live. The next chapter focuses on external things we can do to beat back the darkness, including, in particular, how we care for our physical selves.

And it starts with self-compassion.

Loving Like Jesus

Self-compassion is not just biblical; it's actually foundational to the way Jesus wants us to understand love. Jesus called the instruction to love your neighbor as yourself the second-greatest commandment. In the eyes of Christ, this is second only to loving the Lord with our whole beings. In fact, it's important enough that it made its way into three of the four gospels (Matthew 22:35–40; Mark 12:28–31; Luke 10:25–28).

The word for love here is a deep, broad word that teachers often refer to as God's love. It includes care, compassion, approval, affectionate treatment, and delight. It also carries a sense of a deliberate choice; this type of love is more than just a feeling, but a commitment to seek the welfare of the beloved.[1]

It seems that Jesus actually assumes we will love ourselves like this; if he didn't, he wouldn't have used it as an example for how to love others. He relies on the kind of compassionate care we should have for ourselves to be the model we use to extend love to others. Between a culture that's skilled in tearing us down and the lies of mental illness, that compassionate care doesn't come so naturally to us.

But that's not our fate, friend. As dearly loved children of God, we aren't to be conformed to the patterns of this world. We have the power of the Holy Spirit to help renew our minds and believe the better, truer things that are God's will for us (Romans 12:2).

And those things are rich and beautiful. Isaiah 30:18 (NIV) says that the Lord "longs to be gracious to you; therefore he will rise up to show you compassion." Romans 8:1 tells us there is no condemnation or guilty verdict for those who are in Christ, so we don't have to listen to the critical voice that's so quick to condemn. Instead, as we become more like Jesus, we can look to the biblical instructions on how to love and treat others—as well as the rich, generous ways the Lord loves us—and also apply them to ourselves. Here are a few favorites:

"Speak the truth in love"—even to yourself. (Ephesians 4:15, NLT)

"Don't use foul or abusive language [about yourself]. Let everything you say be good and helpful, so that your words will be an encouragement to those who hear them"—including you. (Ephesians 4:29, NLT)

"Clothe yourselves with compassion, kindness, humility, gentleness and patience." (Colossians 3:12, NIV)

"Forgive [yourself] as the Lord forgave you." (Colossians 3:13, NIV)

"The LORD is good to everyone. He showers compassion on all his creation"—including you. (Psalm 145:9, NLT)

"Rejoice with those who rejoice, weep with those who weep"— not harshly judging our emotions and experiences, but sitting compassionately with our feelings. (Romans 12:15)

The Science of Self-Compassion

There is a ton of scientific support for treating ourselves kindly. Harvard Health has found that it can improve our health, relationships, and overall well-being. It also decreases symptoms of depression and anxiety. As we recognize our own suffering and respond with gentleness, we actually start to feel better.[2]

Our bodies respond to emotional attacks in the same way we respond to physical attacks: by releasing stress hormones and activating the fight-flight-freeze response. This happens whether the attack comes from another person or from inside our own minds. On the flip side, when we intentionally treat ourselves with kindness, we activate the body's soothing and healing response. Instead of stress hormones, we release hormones associated with love, care, and bonding—the same hormones involved in breastfeeding and cuddling.[3]

Licensed therapist Aundi Kolber wrote that extending compassion to ourselves strengthens our internal sense of security, calms our nervous systems, and allows us to access the love and acceptance we so deeply need. While the shaming voice of our inner critics is incapable of producing lasting change, self-compassion and love create true growth and healing. This way, we can reconnect the wounded, broken parts of ourselves through Christlike love and gentleness.[4]

How to Beat Back the Darkness: Getting Practical

At this point, you might be thinking all this sounds great, but it's going to be hard to change the way you think and talk to yourself. That's okay. The good news is that treating yourself kindly is a learnable skill, like all the other ones we've discussed in this book.

Martin Luther once said, "You cannot keep birds from flying over your head, but you can keep them from building a nest in your hair."[5] In other words, thoughts come and go. We can't stop thoughts from popping into our minds. But we can prevent them from making a home there.

Before we get started, there's something we need to remember: these are skills that can be learned. That means that they take practice, they won't come naturally at first, and for a while it will feel like a lot of work. That's okay and normal. It doesn't mean you're doing anything wrong or that it will always feel this difficult.

There will be moments in this process where you feel discouraged and tired of fighting the war in your head. In the middle of the fight, it seems like it's going to last forever. Take courage, friend; as with any skill, it gets easier. Remember, neuroscience is revealing that we can literally rewire our brains over time, so stick with it. Eventually, those new pathways will become well-worn grooves in your mind and it will be so much easier to catch those cruel, toxic thoughts and replace them with kinder, truer words.

There are many books out there on managing our thought lives. You can dive deep on this topic, and honestly, it may be one of the best studies you could do for long-term growth and mental health. But it doesn't have to be complicated. For now, I want to get you started with the practices that have worked for me time and time again.

Mindfulness: Noticing and Detaching

Your thoughts are not you; they're part of what your mind is made to do, just like your lungs are made to breathe and your heart is made to pump blood through your veins. Thoughts rush through our minds constantly; most of the time, we don't even notice them. They create the mental and emotional soundtrack to our lives. Just like the same scene in a movie can seem suspenseful, tender, sad, or funny based on the accompanying music, the thoughts in our heads determine how we interpret and feel about the situations we encounter.

Here's the problem: the thoughts that go through our minds are not all trustworthy and true. We know this because we often experience fears of things that never happen. There was a time when I had a great deal of anxiety about flying. Several times I was certain the plane was going to crash and I would never see Micah again. Of course, those thoughts were not based in reality. It may seem like a silly illustration, but our thoughts about other things—our abilities and value, people's motives, how God feels about us, and what life *should* look like—can be just as untrustworthy.

Thoughts that say life is always going to be this way are untrustworthy. Thoughts that tell you to hurt or kill yourself are extremely untrustworthy. They're telling you that's the only way to get the pain to stop, but they haven't seen the future. There's no way they can know. They're lying to you.

Start by paying attention to your thoughts. When I'm feeling depressed or anxious, I try to listen to my thoughts, almost like I'm eavesdropping on a conversation. That helps me detach a little and observe the things that float through my mind. Then I can remember they're not true; they're just symptoms of depression, anxiety, or trauma.

As you detach from your thoughts, you might find yourself surprised at their content. *I would never say that about another person,* you might realize, or *I'm making assumptions that I don't know are true.* This part might be a little discouraging as you realize how hurtful your thoughts actually are. You might feel like there's no hope to change them, but by paying attention to them, you've already started the process.

Talk Back to the Thoughts

The key to self-compassion is treating yourself the way you'd treat a precious loved one. It really is that simple. And honestly, this is the most important step for me.

I don't have kids, so I imagine I'm talking to one of my nieces, whom I absolutely adore. I think about how I would feel if I heard my sweet seven-year-old niece beating herself up. This helps me connect with the sadness of hearing a loved one treat herself that way. I imagine what I would say to her. Then I tell myself those same things.

For me, it's most effective to say it out loud. It might sound like "You're doing the best you can. It's okay to make mistakes. You're not a bad person," or "Things might feel uncertain right now, but uncertain doesn't mean bad. You're strong and brave, and you've gotten through hard things before. You can do this too."

If talking to yourself doesn't seem to help, try writing yourself a letter. I've written to my younger self about hard times, acknowledging difficult emotions and reminding myself of good things that came after that hard season. You can also imagine you're writing a letter from the future and share the wisdom, hope, and encouragement your imaginary future self might have to offer. The important thing is to find ways to encourage yourself. Say things like:

- *You're going to get through this.*
- *Some of the things you'll learn from this situation are . . .*
- *You can't see it now, but something good that will happen after this is . . .*

Replace the Thought

I've never been able to stop thinking about something by sheer force of will. As soon as I tell myself, *Stop thinking about that,* it's like the thought grows talons and digs in deeper. I've learned it's much more effective to shift my focus to something else.

It's important to know this isn't about denial or pretending the hard, dark feelings aren't there. Instead, it's an intentional choice to turn our attention to something true and beautiful to break the negative loop.

I'll often create lists in my journal of my favorite comforting Bible verses, times God has come through for me, or even times I've been scared or thought I'd messed up but I actually did a good job.

4/30/16

What does my heart need to hear?

Its going to be okay. You don't have to have the answers or a plan or control over this. Yes, self-control is a fruit of the Spirit, but you don't have to have everything figured out. You can be a mess.

Commit to the process. It will probably take longer than you think, but that's okay. If it wasn't a big deal, it would be a shorter process. You'll get there. You really will. What's more is that the Lord has brought you here so far. He's been your help + won't abandon you now.

You're doing a good job. You are doing well. All the paths of the Lord are full of love + faithfulness for you.

There is so much love + grace ahead. Life is not done surprising you - there's plenty more to come. And you are loved dearly, by good friends + by God. You are not alone. You're going to make it.

I also keep a list of those favorite verses and phrases from Scripture on a Pinterest board so they're easily accessible. There have been many times I've breathed through the storm of a panic attack by reading words that are beautiful and true out loud to myself. Here are some of my favorites:

"When my anxious thoughts multiply within me, Your consolations delight my soul." (Psalm 94:19, NASB)

"All the paths of the LORD are steadfast love and faithfulness, for those who keep his covenant and his testimonies." (Psalm 25:10)

"I will never leave you nor forsake you." (Joshua 1:5, NIV)

"You are the God who sees me." (Genesis 16:13, NLT)

"Though I sit in darkness, the LORD will be my light." (Micah 7:8, NLT)

"My flesh and my heart may fail, but God is the strength of my heart and my portion forever." (Psalm 73:26)

"When I am afraid, I will put my trust in you." (Psalm 56:3, NLT)

"He restores my soul." (Psalm 23:3)

"When you pass through the waters, I will be with you; and through the rivers, they shall not overwhelm you; when you walk through fire you shall not be burned, and the flame shall not consume you." (Isaiah 43:2)

"The LORD is near to the brokenhearted and saves the crushed in spirit." (Psalm 34:18)

"The LORD is near to all who call on him." (Psalm 145:18)

Another great option is to listen to music that reminds you of the love of God. There have been many times I've clung to songs that remind me of the closeness and kindness of Immanuel, playing them on repeat and singing their words to my own weary heart.

Worship music can be an obvious choice, but anything that's comforting, encouraging, or hope filled will do.

Build a Gratitude Practice

I used to hate when people would tell me to be more grateful and to "choose joy." *How am I supposed to be thankful for all this pain and this messed-up life? How can I flip a switch and feel better?* They just seemed like more ways I was a bad Christian. I now know these ideas are misunderstandings.

First, the words "choose joy" are not found anywhere in the Bible because we can't simply decide what emotions we will experience. Christians often try to redefine joy by saying it isn't a feeling, but every instance of the word *joy* in Scripture is defined emotionally (gladness, happiness, and mirth are common definitions).[6] So, while it's not possible for me to choose to feel joy, it is possible for me to do things that help cultivate joy in my life. Similarly, Scripture doesn't command us to give thanks for all circumstances. Instead, 1 Thessalonians 5:18 tells us to "give thanks *in* all circumstances."

These are important distinctions. I don't have to be grateful for severe depression, traumatic events, or panic attacks. There's no biblical imperative to thank God for the broken effects of a fallen, sin-sick world. I don't have to try to will myself to feel some fake joy when I'm hurting. But even in the midst of the most horrible moments, there are countless tiny, beautiful things to give thanks for and remembering them helps me cultivate joy bit by bit. So, when I really need to beat back the darkness, I start listing them.

If you saw my gratitude lists, you'd probably be struck at how mundane and simple many of the items are. The bright taste of a tangerine. The warmth of a cup of tea in my hand. A funny text that made me smile. A few minutes FaceTiming with my nieces. A soft hoodie. Anything good in my life—no matter how small or seemingly insignificant—can make the list. And I'll keep writing down everything I can think of, even if I repeat myself day after day.

This is how I've learned to plant and nurture seeds of joy in any

Gratitude
- My snuggly pink sweater
- Funny texts of things my nieces say
- And seeing them on Face Time ♥
- Counseling today
- Micah made me eggs + cinnamon tea for breakfast
- Air conditioning + heat
- That ridiculous inflatable unicorn for Steve
- Favorite children's stories – Pooh + Peter Pan + The Little Prince
- Beautiful, sunny weather
- A perfect walk at the park yesterday
- Comfy pj's
- Fireflies (didn't have them where I grew up - they're so magical!)
- Morning snuggles w/ Micah ♥
- Pens + journals + craft supplies
- That photo of me + my sister
- Blooming trees
- Fresh coffee
- Texts from friends ♥

and every season—even the darkest depressive episodes. This habit is threaded all throughout Scripture, and for good reason: intentionally expressing thanks helps us pause and see the goodness of God in our lives.

We learn to see more of God's gifts as we appreciate them. As we see more goodness in this life, our hearts can't help but expand with joy, though it may be more accurate to say our neural circuits rewire over time. A seismic shift in perspective and our capacity for joy starts in this tiny habit.

That's why verses like Psalms 30:11–12 and 9:1 say, "I will give thanks to you forever" or "with my whole heart." God doesn't *need* our gratitude or praise; our hearts need to express gratitude to him in order to experience the truest joy.

Talk About It

Sometimes, you can do all the right things on your own but you just need somebody. Beating back the darkness is about moving toward better health—and in our darkest moments, that means doing whatever is necessary to keep ourselves safe. I've found that if I tell somebody I'm struggling with dark thoughts, it's much less tempting to act on them.

When fear and stigma told me to keep silent about thoughts of suicide and self-harm, I reached out to safe, supportive people for accountability. Every time I had thoughts of self-harm or suicide in a counseling session, I would simply mention them to my therapist. If I wasn't in therapy, I would text a good friend who I knew wouldn't judge me. It's usually not necessary or helpful to be graphic; just saying the thoughts were coming into my mind took a lot of power out of them. They didn't seem so convincing then.

It helps to have a conversation with your safe people to explain what you experience and how they can help you stay safe. You might say something like "One of the symptoms of severe depression is having thoughts of self-harm or suicide. I experience that sometimes. I don't really want to hurt myself, but it would help me stay safe if I could share when those thoughts come up." You can also work with your counselor to come up with a way to talk to friends and family that works for you.

Also, please be honest with yourself and your loved ones. Sometimes, the thoughts become too intense and we need some extra help to get better. If you don't feel like you can commit to staying safe, or you find yourself actively making plans for a suicide attempt, ask somebody to stay with you and, if necessary, help you get to a hospital.

When I was first learning to fight against the thoughts, the temptation to self-harm was ferocious. I often texted my friends Steve and Lindsey, but there were times the thoughts were too loud and I didn't know if I could resist on my own. Steve and Lindsey told me to get my butt in the car and head over to their house. So I did, even though they live three hours away. Driving to Birmingham seemed extreme, but I was learning to believe I'm worth whatever it takes to stay safe and get better.

Those thoughts aren't so common for me anymore, but they do come around occasionally. I'm still committed to telling somebody when thoughts of hurting myself intrude on my mind, because I refuse to allow them to grow in the darkness of shame and secrecy. Usually, I tell my husband, Micah, something simple and direct, like "I've been having thoughts of self-harm." But I've also come up with code words to use with friends when it feels too tough to speak so plainly. Either way, it's never a fun conversation to have, but I am always grateful to be able to have it because it helps keep me safe.

I know this stuff isn't easy, and the changes don't happen nearly as quickly as we'd prefer. When you're deeply depressed and dark thoughts are assaulting you from every angle, it's natural to feel overwhelmed and frozen. It takes a lot of energy to constantly turn our attention back to what is beautiful and true, to catch the negative thoughts we think about ourselves and speak kindly instead.

That's okay. It's perfectly normal. If we've been in the pit for a while, we've built up habits that keep us embedded in our own pain. Now we have the opportunity to build new habits, create new patterns, and help our brains rewire for joy and hope, even in the midst of depression. It takes time and it won't happen overnight. But it can happen, my friend. Keep at it. You can learn to beat back the darkness.

Fifteen

Ruthless with Self-Care

The rule was this: if I didn't feel worth it, I had to do it. It didn't matter if "it" was cooking a healthy meal or buying myself flowers. It didn't matter if it was making myself a chai or spending time with my sketchbook. What did matter was that I fought back against the belief that I was not worth getting better.

I'm not entirely sure how I came up with the rule. I think it just occurred to me at one point after a therapy session when I realized how little I like to take care of myself. I looked around my apartment and saw piles of laundry, bare walls because I hadn't made the effort to decorate, and a nearly empty fridge.

So I bought myself flowers. Every week after therapy I went to the grocery store and picked a bundle or two, fresh and bright and cheerful, to remind me that I am alive. I pulled the one chair I owned onto my tiny concrete patio and slowly sipped my chai in the cool of the morning. I found the energy to cook and pack healthier lunches even when it didn't seem worth the effort because I didn't seem worth the effort.

I began to treat myself like I mattered. I began to treat myself as though I had value. And eventually, it started to sink in. I started to believe that I wasn't so bad after all.

When weariness seemed to gnaw at my bones, I took a gentle walk just to see the sun. I stopped at an empty playground and sat on the swings, slowly pumping my legs and remembering how I used to imagine I could fly. I lay on a picnic table, stared up into the blue expanse, tried to soak the life and light back into my being.

I didn't feel like it.

I didn't believe it would help.

I wasn't sure I even *wanted* to believe I could get better.

I did it anyway.

———

It's easy to go through life and never examine what you *really* believe. You don't question the whispers in your head and the feelings in your chest—certainly everyone else experiences life the same way, right?

I always thought everyone was hard on themselves like I am, with high internal standards and constant pressure to meet them. For years, I failed to recognize, much less question, the quiet sense of shame that pervaded my soul. It was a simple reality to me: *I am not good enough.*

Therapy helped me unearth that belief; I started to work on it as I learned to speak kindly to myself. Still, I found I needed more than just gentle and kind words. I needed to behave as if I mattered, as if I was worthy of kind treatment. The best way I could do that was to change the way I treated my body.

So I became ruthless with self-care. *Ruthless* may seem like a strange word to apply to self-care, but in retrospect, it seems like the best way to describe the mental shift I made.

After all, mental illness is a cruel beast, brutal and bold, insidious and sneaky. The worst moments creep up and pounce on you with all the stealth and ferocity of a wildcat. You can be just fine, when suddenly the clouds roll in—quick and violent like a storm, or gradual and quiet, like a fog. Either way, you find yourself in the midst of it and suddenly you're drowning. Suddenly there is no air, your chest hurts from trying to breathe, and you can't see which way is up. It lies constantly, says you're worthless, and doesn't care if you need a respite.

Over the past few years, we've lost a lot of faith leaders to suicide. It's always jarring and disorienting to read the headlines. My heart breaks, thinking about the families and friends grieving such a shattering loss. My head also spins because many of these people have spoken out about the darkness, been open about their struggles, and advocated to destigmatize mental illness, just like me.

Many were deeply cared for and supported well by loved ones. Some were under the care of doctors and therapists and wrestled in the dark for many years, while others experienced a sudden and terrifying plunge into the pit, scarcely having time to catch their breath and learn to manage their conditions. We cannot possibly judge the final moments of those who die from mental illness because we can't know all the details of their private battles against a ferocious disease.

It's scary to see those we look up to die by suicide, especially when they look just like us. But we can honor their lives and messages by allowing them to spur us on in our own fights. My dear friend, we can't afford to give mental illness an inch. We can't get complacent or assume we're past these struggles.

If this unyielding illness can steal the lives of even those who publicly fight against it, we have to fight back just as ferociously. We must be just as merciless against depression and thoughts of suicide as they are against us.

This is why we must be ruthless with self-care and our fight for wholeness. This is why, as my friend Blake once said, we must decide on our good days who we will be on our bad days. We put plans in place to care for ourselves, body and brain and soul, to push back the howling ache and keep it from robbing us of our lives too.

Put in this light, self-care becomes a nonnegotiable. The things I do to take care of myself in my bad seasons keep me back from the ledge where I toy with the idea of ending my life. And the things I do to take care of myself in my better seasons set me up for success and keep me healthier overall.

What Is Self-Care?

Self-care is a buzzword that shows up in all our Instagram feeds. But it's not coffee cups, bubble baths, and scented candles. It's much more like parenting a beloved child.

In *Miracles and Other Reasonable Things,* Sarah Bessey shares an insight from a friend about the difference between self-care and self-comfort. When we say self-care, we're usually picturing something more akin to self-comfort: soothing pedicures, reading a relaxing book, snuggling up under a warm blanket and watching a fun show.[1]

All those things are wonderful and can be important ways to love ourselves. Being able to comfort ourselves is important, especially when we're flooded with emotions and need to be able to calm down. It's a component of self-care, but it's not all of it, because self-comfort is focused on the immediate need. It's what we do when we feel stressed, anxious, or depressed and take some immediate actions to help ourselves feel better.

Self-care also focuses on the long term. It's not just the instant need of self-comfort, but the future-focused perspective of needs that are inevitable. This is why it's like parenting a beloved child. A "good parent"[2] balances both immediate needs and the growth of the child into a whole, healthy adult. So Mom kisses the scrapes and Dad holds the crying child, but they also make sure the vegetables get eaten. They make sure the kid goes outside to play. They take the child for checkups and vaccinations and teach him life lessons. This way, the parent helps build a bright future for a healthy, resilient child.

Obviously, not every parent is healthy. Not every parent knows what she's doing or is good at parenting. But in a stable, functional home, this is what care for a child looks like. Even if we didn't grow up in healthy, functional homes where we experienced good care most of the time, we can learn to care for ourselves in a healthy way. We can start taking care of both the immediate needs and the long-term goals. And over time, we learn that this is how God wants to take care of us too.

It's easy to compromise on what we need when culture tells us the path to well-being is anything from hustling our faces off (*I'll sleep when I'm dead!*) to doing whatever feels good in the moment. The problem with both of those views is that they don't take a holistic perspective of caring for ourselves. Sometimes, we have to work hard for periods of time. Sometimes, we need to rest and take a break. Sometimes, a treat is fine, and other times we need to eat vegetables because managing our blood sugar helps our moods stay steadier and we don't get anxious.

When we're severely depressed, we often struggle with healthy self-care: not eating or sleeping healthy amounts, for example, or not getting out of the house to see the sun for days on end. Sometimes, these challenges are due to some of the physical symptoms of depression. Fatigue and lack of energy make it tough to find motivation.

Other times, it's due to the dark thoughts and lies we believe about ourselves that come with depression. I struggled to value myself. I couldn't see the image of God staring back at me in the mirror so I couldn't find a reason to care for myself. For many of us in the dark, it may be easier to see the image of God in other people than in ourselves.

Depression happens in the body, not just the soul and psyche. It's not this ethereal thing, unmoored from physicality. It's gritty and earthy, if still not fully understood, woven into the pathways that course through our tissues.

That's where I worked out its effects, in self-harm and lack of self-care, in sleepless nights and days I couldn't get out of bed, in plans to sever the connection between soul and body because I couldn't bear to inhabit my skin anymore.

When we skip meals or binge eat to manage the emotions, we're trying to control an illness that happens in the body. When we cry and when our hearts race, when our stomachs ache and our breathing feels labored, our bodies are sending signals about our health.

It's funny that we call it mental health. It surely affects our minds, our thought patterns, and our emotions. But all those things are so interconnected with our bodies that it's almost laughable to ignore the rest of the equation. The symptoms that often lead us to our doctors aren't that we feel sad, but the chest pain, nausea and acid reflux, extreme fatigue or unshakeable insomnia.

Those symptoms are signals that something is wrong and we need to take care of ourselves; that means taking care of our bodies. And taking care of our bodies results in tangible changes in the way our brains and bodies work.

Nourish and Cherish Yourself

As we saw in the last chapter, Scripture tells us to "love your neighbor as yourself," assuming some basic level of care (Matthew 22:39; Mark 12:31; Luke 10:27). In other words, Jesus expects us to love ourselves. In Ephesians, when given the example of how to love and care for our spouses, it says husbands should love their wives as their own bodies because "no one ever hated his own flesh, but nourishes and cherishes it" (Ephesians 5:28–29).

Those of us who struggle with depression may not be very good at nourishing and cherishing our bodies. But even in this, Jesus sets an example for us; his life demonstrated a lot of healthy self-care habits. Jesus listened to his body and was kind to it, treating it with the respect due an "earthly temple." He took walks and naps, ate well, and went to social gatherings to spend time with friends and family (Mark 1:16; 4:38; Luke 5:33; 7:34; John 12:2).

First Corinthians 6:19–20 tells us that our bodies are the temple of the Holy Spirit who lives within us. In the verse, Paul charged us to honor God with our bodies. Though the original context was about sexual integrity, the principle can be applied to anything else we do with our bodies—eating, sleeping, exercising, and so on.

More than Just Mental

While some streams of thought about severe depression focus solely on the brain (looking at genetic factors or talking about chemical imbalances, for example) and others look at the role of the mind (our thought patterns and mental habits), new research is revealing that there's another huge piece of the puzzle: our bodies as whole, integrated systems. Edward Bullmore, author of *The Inflamed Mind: A Radical New Approach to Depression,* argued that it's time to "move on from the old polarised view of depression as all in the mind or all in the brain to see it as rooted also in the body." He went on to say that we need to see depression instead as a way our bodies respond to the difficulties of surviving in a hostile world.[3]

In other words, this raging darkness isn't just about negative thoughts or a lack of serotonin. It's about our whole lives, our whole bodies, and our whole selves. And that means that everything we do has the potential to impact our mental health. This is a big deal because it means there are countless things we can adjust in our lives to feel better and we have much more control over our illnesses than was previously understood. Treatment isn't limited to a pill or therapy session; it happens every day as we eat, sleep, interact with others, and move our bodies.

That's why genuine self-care is absolutely crucial if we want to live well despite the darkness. Some of us may not be able to completely cure our depression, but what if we could turn down the intensity by 60, 70, 80 percent? What if, even when you noticed the spiraling thoughts starting, you had some simple practices that could help your body feel calm, safe, and soothed? That's what a holistic self-care plan that integrates taking care of our bodies does.

This might seem absurd, but research is emerging that shows inflammation causes depressive symptoms and behaviors in both animals and people. Why would our bodies do this? Well, inflammation is part of an immune system response—it happens when our bodies are fighting off some sort of an intruder that could make us ill. One of the hallmarks of depression is that feeling of exhaustion that can drive you to bed, just like when you have the flu. Basically, it's your immune system's way of trying to get you to rest so it can more efficiently fight off infection.[4]

Part of me is awestruck by this research; it reveals another wonderfully complex way God designed our bodies to take care of us. And it makes perfect sense that we would benefit from a brief period of rest to get over an illness.

But what if inflammation becomes chronic, our immune systems battling constantly? It makes sense that depression could become chronic too. Research is confirming this through links between mental illnesses and autoimmune disorders.[5] While scientists are unearthing connections between mental health and physical processes in the body, that information hasn't yet translated into new clinical treatments for contributing factors like inflammation.[6]

We've all heard the advice to eat right, sleep well, and get some exercise. We *know* those are important elements of self-care and that those things are good for all living creatures. Some of us have even been told that these changes are "all we need" to start feeling better. It's more complicated than that, to be sure, and most of us won't entirely eradicate the darkness by eating some salad and going for a run. But we do need to take these lifestyle changes seriously. Because we're learning that our lifestyles have a huge impact on the way our bodies work—like through stress hormones that increase inflammation.

Of course, inflammation isn't the whole story. We know now that depression—and mental illness in general—is linked to many factors, so we need to let go of the idea that there is any single cure-all for our illnesses.[7] Still, there is mounting evidence that we can powerfully manage our symptoms when we practice good self-care over time. Dr. Alex Korb explains it this way: "Feeling better is simply a combination of finding the right life changes for you to create the right brain changes. Everyone's brain is different, and everyone's depression is different, so treatment is often an exploration."[8]

The great news is that there are many, many options to explore. Most of these options also have a significant impact on overall health, which is especially important as those with mental health diagnoses have a shorter life expectancy than the general population by ten to twenty years. This is primarily due to physical chronic diseases that often result from a lack of good self-care.[9]

Fueling Mental Wellness

A small study of the impact of diet in mental illness found that 32 percent of participants experienced complete remission from their depression after twelve weeks. This study used a modified Mediterranean diet and focused on getting participants to eat balanced, whole-food diets. The recommended diet was rich in whole grains, vegetables, fruits, balanced protein sources (eggs, lean meats, and fish), and healthy fats (olive oil and nuts), while limiting processed, fried, or fast foods, sweets or sugary drinks, and refined cereals.[10]

I didn't seriously look at my diet until Micah started noticing that I often became anxious, panicked, or more depressed when it had been too long since I'd eaten a healthy meal. As I started paying attention, it became clear that my sugar intake seriously impacted my mental health symptoms. I'd also gained forty pounds in the first year I was on antidepressants, my stomach often hurt, and I was getting near-constant migraines.

Some research led me to try a modified Paleo diet (which I now know is similar to the plan from the above study) for thirty days, sure it would be a short experiment and that I would go back to my normal habits. After about ten days (once I was past the sugar cravings), I realized the several-times-a-week panic attacks had stopped. Much of the fatigue I'd attributed to depression dissipated, my stomach stopped hurting, and I generally felt more calm and even.

That thirty-day experiment happened three years ago, and I haven't gone back. I lost most of the weight I'd gained, I have far fewer headaches (though that's still an issue for me), and I have full-blown panic attacks only every few months now. I never would have imagined that what I eat would make such a difference in my mental health.

When depression makes us feel exhausted, overwhelmed, or apathetic, it's tough to find the motivation to cook healthy meals, but there are ways to make it easier on yourself. First, pay attention to how your body responds to different foods. For me, refined sugar and processed carbohydrates (white bread, for example) wreak havoc on my anxiety. I may take a couple of bites of Micah's dessert and be fine, but I know that if I eat an entire piece of birthday cake, I'll feel panicky and depressed later.

Next, find some go-to foods that are easy and don't take much effort. For me, those are smoothies (just throw ingredients in a blender), scrambled eggs with veggies (takes less time than it takes to make a box of mac 'n' cheese), plain Greek yogurt with berries and seeds, and an apple with almond butter. Micah and I also like to meal plan to save the energy of trying to figure out what to make. When we can, we cook large portions of healthy meals (using a slow cooker or pressure cooker to make it easy) so there are lots of leftovers, freezing whatever we won't eat before it spoils.

Moving Our Bodies

I know you've heard this, friend. And if you're anything like me, you hate to hear it again. Because the crushing fatigue and intense lack of motivation make it seem next to impossible to lace up your shoes and head to the gym. This is the one I struggle with the most, partly because chronic pain makes it tough to participate in the exercises I used to love. Since so many people with mental illness also have other chronic diagnoses, that adds another layer of difficulty in getting our bodies moving.

But this is an area I've learned I have to be ruthless about in my self-care because it really does help. Exercise profoundly changes how our brains and bodies work, just like antidepressants do. Exercise increases serotonin and dopamine (neurotransmitters targeted by antidepressants) and helps repair parts of the brain related to learning and memory that shrink during depression. Studies have shown that as little as thirty minutes of brisk walking three times per week can be as effective as medication for some patients.[11] One small study found that after ten months, those who continued to walk three times per week were much more likely to be free of depressive symptoms than those who were on antidepressants.[12]

It's utterly crucial that the exercise be something you enjoy. When we're struggling to function, it's next to impossible to go to the gym for a grueling, miserable workout. But finding something enjoyable or purposeful is much easier to participate in. It's also important to get your heart rate up a little. You can tell you're in the ideal intensity range if it's a little harder to carry on a conversation (your sentences become a little choppy) but you're not gasping for breath.[13]

I have found a few things that work well for me on good days and bad. Micah and I walk together a few times each week, and he often reminds me I need to move when I'm in a tough season. I also love to work out in the pool, even on dark days; the cool water is soothing, it's gentle on my joints, and I can get a decent aerobic workout without feeling like I'm working too hard.

Finally, set your expectations low to start. I've found this to be key to starting almost any habit in my life. It's important to feel like we're achieving a goal, especially when we don't feel like we can achieve much of anything. When I was getting used to working out at the pool in a tough depression season, my only goal was to get into the water. Once I did that, I counted it a win (plus, at that point, it's easier to spend some time working out than it is to just turn around and go home). Low expectations can be a sneaky way to accomplish much more.

(Note that if you deal with any type of eating disorder, please make sure you work with your team of professionals to find out what is safe and healthy for you. While exercise can be a powerful way to manage depression, if done excessively, it can also reinforce dangerous habits for those with eating disorders. Please take good care of yourself.)

Stress Management and Feeling Safe

"My body is the home that holds me," Aundi Kolber wrote. "And how can we grow and change if we can't feel at peace in our homes? Physiologically, how can we process and learn if we don't feel safe with ourselves?"[14]

Stress and anxiety are the result of feeling unsafe or threatened in some way. They are God-given messengers telling us something is wrong and we need to be alert and ready to outrun, outfight, or freeze to outwit an attacker.

Trauma, particularly abuse, teaches us our bodies aren't safe places to be, that painful and scary things can happen to them. This might leave us with a sense of our bodies' failing or betraying us, or a belief that our bodies are intrinsically bad or shameful.[15] These beliefs become embedded in our implicit memories and become coping mechanisms, designed to keep us safe from further pain.[16]

But none of those things are helpful when we're only wrestling internally, not fighting something outside ourselves. We need ways to manage stress that let our bodies and brains know we're safe.

In *The Body Keeps the Score,* a landmark book that explains how trauma changes us and how to treat it, Dr. Bessel van der Kolk explored how we can find a sense of safety in our bodies. For some patients who didn't respond to traditional counseling, things like massage therapy helped them come home to their bodies and feel at peace in them.[17] Through his work with patients experiencing mental illness and particularly trauma, he discovered we must *befriend* our bodies and their sensations to find healing.[18]

One way to do this is through mindful physical movement, like gentle stretching exercises or light strength work. Another option is yoga, if you feel comfortable practicing it in light of its physical benefits—it can be an effective way to manage stress and create a sense of security in your body. I've found it incredibly helpful. The simple combination of breathing exercises, focused attention, and moving through poses positively impacts depression, anxiety, and anger, as well as being very healing for those with PTSD.[19] It increases awareness of what's going on in our bodies, which is crucial for good self-care. After all, if we don't know what our bodies need, we can't respond to those needs as a loving parent would.[20]

While calm stretching can feel great and reduce stress, any movement that brings you into the present moment can help. Some people may find dance or martial arts to be good ways to connect with your body. Whatever exercise you choose, remember to balance learning to sit with discomfort and not pushing too hard or trying to compete with others.

Do Something You (Used to) Love

One of the hallmark symptoms of depression is a lack of enjoyment or pleasure in activities that we previously enjoyed. We may have relished tending a garden, trying new recipes, or practicing calligraphy, but it seems like all the fun has seeped right out. Combined with the fatigue and lack of motivation, this can make it tough to pursue a new pastime (or even an old one) during a depressive episode.

Taking up a hobby is linked to reducing symptoms of depression as well as reducing by 30 percent the risk of developing depression. Those who started a hobby after already being depressed experienced a staggering 272 percent higher odds of recovering from that depression.[21]

Even if you struggle to see the point of your activities or to feel pleasure, be intentional to make time for a hobby that used to fill up your heart. If you don't have one, pick a new one and set low standards as you learn. Over the past few years, I've gotten into watercolor painting by following simple tutorials online (and with a lot of encouragement from my sister, who is an artist herself). I often don't try to accomplish anything or paint a finished piece. Instead, I just enjoy playing with the colors and letting them soothe me.

If you have a hobby already—that thing you think of as your "happy place" or "safe place" when you're feeling good—your body and soul need you to keep doing that thing. If you usually love to cook, try a new recipe. Is music your thing? Take ten minutes to just play something you enjoy without focusing too hard on getting it perfect. It could be gardening, woodworking, arts and crafts, restoring old cars, or something else entirely. It really doesn't matter what it is as long as you would usually find it enjoyable and engrossing.

Sleep

This one can feel so elusive. Simple advice to get some rest doesn't work; many of us know that struggling to sleep the right amount is a common part of depression. We may use sleep as an escape, wake without feeling rested, or toss and turn all night.

Common wisdom is that mental illnesses often cause sleep problems; researchers are learning that the opposite can be true too. This is called a bidirectional effect: sleep problems can cause mental health problems and vice versa.[22] Studies suggest that up to 90 percent of patients with depression have some sort of sleep problem, with insomnia being the most common.[23]

The good news is that many other self-care practices (regular aerobic exercise, good nutrition, and relaxation techniques like mindfulness meditation) can help us sleep better over time. Sleep hygiene can also help; these are habits that train the brain and body to sleep well, like going to bed and getting up at the same time every day, not watching TV or looking at screens in bed, and making sure the bedroom is used "only for sleeping or sex."[24]

I dealt with insomnia, nightmares, and poor sleep for most of my life. Working through past trauma in therapy made a big difference in my sleep patterns but so did developing some bedtime rituals. Every night as I get ready for bed, I stretch a little or massage any tight muscles. Then I lie down and listen to a guided meditation that focuses on intentionally relaxing. Micah and I pray together before bed, which helps me feel like we end the day well. I've also cut out caffeine from the midafternoon on, and I sleep with a fan, ear plugs, and an eye mask. When I really struggle to sleep, I use a weighted blanket (which is also incredibly helpful for anxiety and panic attacks).

If you try all these tips and are still having trouble getting good rest, please talk to your doctor. Underlying conditions such as sleep apnea might be impacting your mental health, for example. Your doctor might have other ideas, like switching the time of day you take medications, trying out supplements like melatonin, or even a short course of sleeping medication to help reset your body's sleep cycle (all of which I've had doctors suggest to me).

Pay Attention to Media Consumption

I love sad songs, suspenseful crime shows, and dramatic movies. For many years, my favorite movie was a film adaptation of *Hamlet,* a tragic story of loss, revenge, suicide, and murder. Watching a heart-breaking movie can be cathartic, but it can also feed depression, while psychological thrillers fuel my anxiety. And of course, many news outlets can be a source of fear, outrage, and pain. So I've learned to be careful about what I watch, read, and listen to, especially if I'm feeling low or anxious.

But media can also be a tool for self-care that helps us reconnect with positive emotions. Funny video clips from late-night shows have gotten me through panic attacks and out of bed on hard days. I unfollow social media accounts that make me feel worse, keep a playlist of cheerful music on my phone for the moments I need a boost, and make time to watch comedies when the clouds are rolling in. Laughter really can be good medicine to help us get through our hard days.

———

Our bodies are a gift to allow us to interact with this brilliant, beautiful world. Fallenness means they don't always work as well as God intended for us to experience, but they are wonderful gifts, nonetheless. Our bodies carry us through life, in all its lovely and terrible moments; they enable us to experience creation, one another, and God himself.

As a dearly loved child of God, you deserve to be treated with dignity and kindness. My friend, that means even your body, and even by yourself. If all these changes seem overwhelming, that's perfectly fine. Just start by looking for ways to incorporate some kindness and nurturing into your days. As that becomes easier, start thinking ahead, making choices on your better days that set you up for success on the darker days.

You are worthy of this. You are worth everything it takes to get better.

Sixteen

Boundaries, Loving Others,
and Soul-Keeping

I don't want to hear that.

When I worked in a residential mental health facility for young women, we used to say the residents didn't come with trigger warnings. Inevitably, staff members had some of our own baggage come up from time to time in working with the young women. Some residents refused to open up. But others would serially over-share traumatic details that were enough to give you nightmares. At the very least, a few stories triggered panic attacks, suicidal thoughts, and self-harm urges in me.

Even though I worked in the mental health field with women who had been severely traumatized, I still had to take care of myself. I was responsible for modeling healthy boundaries for these women; they also needed to know it was okay to say they weren't comfortable discussing something that wasn't healthy for them. I had to learn to say, "That's something to discuss in your counseling session" or invite them to journal about what they were processing.

The time I spent working at the residential facility taught me so much about boundaries. The job was physically and emotionally demanding. I often felt the kind of fatigue that made me wonder if I should be driving home from my shifts because it seemed like being drunk. I had to learn when to say no to going out with friends and take a nap instead, which was a hard balance; sometimes I said no too many times, and sometimes I didn't say it enough.

I *loved* my work. It was fulfilling, rewarding, and life giving, allowing me to walk through really hard stuff with people and help them find healing. But over time, it took a toll. The workplace was imperfect, like all workplaces, and wasn't structured well to support the long-term health of certain roles. When my physical and mental health began to unravel in a stressful job with unhealthy expectations, I realized that I had to better steward my time, energy, and health.

That led me to draw a big boundary: shifting out of traditional ministry and leaving the nonprofit world.

I *agonized* over that decision. I felt like I was abandoning the young women I worked with, letting God down, forsaking my calling, and, frankly, being weak. *I should be strong enough to do my own healing and carry the weight of all these other stories,* I thought. But it didn't work that way. I had to learn that, if I wanted to truly love and serve those God had called me to, I needed to be healthy enough to do it. That meant I needed to step away for a season.

———

I remember when I was first learning about boundaries, a friend used the illustration of a Hula-Hoop. If I have one around my waist, everything I can control is inside that hoop—my actions, my thoughts, my reactions. I can't control what's inside anybody else's hoop.

But what was a revelation to me was that *nobody else was responsible for what's inside my hoop.* You might be thinking that this is obvious—of course nobody else is responsible for my actions, thoughts, beliefs, reactions. What wasn't obvious to me was that I get to take care of myself without waiting for anybody else to take care of me.

My family and church experiences had taught me to put myself last, to never ask for anything, to bend myself to fit the shape that others imagined for me. Somewhere along the way, I grew a belief that I had to wait for somebody else to notice I was struggling and to help me. In my mind, I wasn't allowed to help myself, so I was at the mercy of leaders and loved ones. So I waited for rescue, all the while running my body and brain into the ground.

Of course, nobody came to save me. Not because anyone was bad or selfish. But because nobody reads minds and because I am the only one responsible for myself. So for many people, learning about boundaries is the first time we find ourselves saying no to people. For me, it was one of the first times I said yes to myself.

In *Boundaries* by Henry Cloud and John Townsend, there's an illustration of some parents learning about the importance of "watering their own yard" instead of enabling their son:

> Look at it this way. It is as if he's your neighbor, who never waters his lawn. But whenever you turn on your sprinkler system, the water falls on his lawn. Your grass is turning brown and dying, but Joshua looks down at his green grass and thinks to himself, *My yard is doing fine.* That is how your son's life is. He doesn't study or plan or work, yet he has a nice place to live, plenty of money, and all the rights of a family member who is doing his part.[1]

While I wasn't a parent enabling a drug-addicted son (as in the illustration), I *had* been spending so much time with my sprinkler pointed at everyone else's yard that mine was growing parched and dry. I wanted to be a good Christian and a loving person, so I thought I needed to put everyone else first. But I was dying of thirst, never realizing I had not only the right but the responsibility to turn the sprinkler around onto my own patch of lawn.

Tending a Garden

The Bible opens with a story that sets the stage for all of humanity. Genesis 2:15 tells us that "the LORD God placed the man in the Garden of Eden to tend and watch over it" (NLT). It's a beautiful picture of God creating the first person and giving him this gorgeous garden to care for. In a story that tells us of a perfect world, God gave humankind something precious to watch over. And just like Adam and Eve, we were each given a garden to tend: Our lives. Our souls.

In Proverbs, we're told to keep careful watch over our hearts because they're the source of everything in our lives (Proverbs 4:23). It's another way God tells us he's given us our lives as a gift to care for and cultivate.

I love how Galatians 6:5 in The Message says it: "Each of you must take responsibility for doing the creative best you can with your own life." Other translations talk about being responsible to "bear our own loads." The load described here has to do with a normal, reasonable weight we carry; it's not about something super heavy that would weigh us down too much. (Just a few verses before, in Galatians 6:2, we're told to "share each other's burdens" [NLT]. The word for "burden" describes an excessively heavy weight that's too much for one person to bear.)

Here's the takeaway for us: bearing our own loads means taking care of the everyday things that go on inside us. It means doing what we can to manage our thoughts, our emotions, and our choices because nobody else on earth can carry them for us. It means we get to partner with God to learn to shoulder our loads and walk with him.

It's beautiful that, in this area, as in all others, Jesus is our ultimate example. We know that Jesus came to serve, to love, and to lay his life down. But we might miss the fact that he maintained healthy boundaries throughout his life. In Luke 4:30, Jesus slipped away through the crowd of people who were trying to hurt him (before it was time for him to go to the cross). He also knew when to retreat and prioritize his need for rest (Mark 4:35–40), time alone (Mark 1:35; Matthew 14:13), and even food (John 21:12—I love that right after he rose from the dead, Jesus wanted to have breakfast with his disciples).

Yes, Jesus did exemplify the greatest of loves by laying his life down for us. But he also leaned in, listened to the Father, and knew that he was a valuable and beloved child of God too. He didn't sacrifice every natural desire and need to other people each moment of his life. When it counted, he laid his life down. But he practiced the healthy boundaries he needed to carry himself through his ministry, maintain a healthy relationship with his Father, and accomplish his ultimate mission.

Don't Sacrifice Your Soul

Healthy boundaries can be difficult to implement when they haven't been modeled or accepted for us early in life. Aundi Kolber explained it this way in *Try Softer:*

> When our caregivers continually communicate that we don't have a voice, we may learn it's better just to tell them what they want to hear. Then we carry that perception into adulthood and our relationships with other people. . . . When this is the script we live from, we are likely to mistrust our own instincts and avoid advocating for ourselves.

Kolber wrote that, as we deny our own experiences to appease others, we're not as able to handle the ups and downs of life. We may think we're being "good Christians" and "loving others," but failing to set boundaries actually sacrifices our souls in a way God never intended for us. We need healthy boundaries to help us tend the gardens God has entrusted to us—our very souls. And we certainly need healthy boundaries to live well despite a mental illness diagnosis.[2]

How to Start Setting Boundaries

Setting boundaries can feel impossible because it can generate so many emotions in our bodies. The fear of disappointing or hurting people can make us feel sick with dread or shame, as though taking care of our own needs is horribly selfish.[3] But, my dear friend, those feelings are lying to us. It is not selfish, shameful, or wrong to care for "your one wild and precious life."[4]

Boundaries show up in a million different ways. Here are a handful of ways I've implemented them in my life.

Boundaries with Strangers and Acquaintances

It may be easiest to set boundaries with people you're not close to. The stakes just don't feel as high when you're practicing setting limits. Practically, this might look like a gracious "No, but thank you for asking" when somebody invites you to something you're not interested in or asks for your help with something you don't feel good about committing to.

A friend of mine once shared that she sometimes says "Thank you, but I have a previous commitment" when she is invited to something she doesn't have time or energy for. Her eyes glimmered playfully when she said she had made a commitment to herself not to say yes to things she shouldn't. I do think it's appropriate to be more direct, but if you don't feel you can simply answer "I can't make it" or "I won't be able to," you can borrow her creative response.

Boundaries with Loved Ones

Setting boundaries with loved ones is especially tough at first because none of us want to hurt the people we care for most. But after a while, people generally get used to it. After all, to some extent, we teach people how to treat us. (I'm not saying if somebody treats you poorly, it's your fault. I am saying that, based on what we tolerate and what consequences and results come from how people treat us, they learn what we're okay with and treat us accordingly.)

For example, I absolutely love visiting my sister and her family. I adore spending time with them, playing with the kids, and want to squeeze every moment of quality time out of every visit. On the other hand, I'm an introvert and I will not be a kind, healthy person if I don't get time to myself. This led to a few frustrating visits when I found myself exhausted, "peopled out," and yet afraid to ask for some time alone. I realized if I wanted to enjoy the time together, I needed to take care of myself. So my sister and I figured out some options, like making sure I had access to a vehicle, and we both understood I would go take some alone time. During one visit, Micah and I left the family festivities on Christmas afternoon to take a nap before dinner.

Other boundaries I've learned to implement include:

- not answering the phone or texts right away
- removing myself from unhealthy situations
- setting expectations in advance (for example, if I can stay at a gathering for only one hour)

Boundaries with Yourself

Internal boundaries are the ones we establish for ourselves and can be a kind way to practice self-care. My therapist recently told me that setting limits with ourselves allows us to accept ourselves as we are, not as we wish we were. As we come to know who we are and what works for us, we are able to set compassionate boundaries that help us live happier, healthier lives.

Social media can be terrible for my mental health and my productivity. Sure, I've made great connections and built incredible friendships online, and this book wouldn't exist if it weren't for an article I wrote getting shared on Facebook. But it's far too easy for me to lose time doomscrolling and lose peace to the vitriol so common in my feed. I'm tempted to think that shouldn't bother me or I just shouldn't go to those sites, but the simple reality is it does bother me and those sites are legitimately addictive. Instead of beating myself up, I needed to find loving ways to set myself up for success.

In this case, setting boundaries with myself means using tools that help me avoid the unhealthy aspects of social media. I've installed apps on my computer and phone browsers that block my Facebook feed (called Feedless for iPhone and Feed Eradicator for Google Chrome); I can still share updates or go to private groups, but I'm not bombarded with posts that fuel anger or stress. I don't keep social media apps installed on my phone because it's too easy to mindlessly click on them when I'm bored. I also keep notifications turned off for everything except calls and texts. And when I've got a writing deadline and I can't afford to waste time, I ask Micah to change my social media passwords for me.

In the past, I would have beaten myself up for not being "strong enough" or having the willpower to make things work a different way. Aundi Kolber calls this white-knuckling, and it can show up so many different ways. I've tried to will myself to keep my emotions in check, to power through when I've needed to rest, to keep saying yes when my body and soul are screaming for me to say no.

Boundaries are often the remedy to white-knuckling. In fact, one of the most life-giving lessons I learned in my journey to thriving despite severe depression was how to live with healthy limits. Yes, it often felt excruciating, like I was constantly letting somebody down and should just be strong enough to handle it all. But it was so worth it to learn to advocate for myself like this. I couldn't have foreseen that the boundaries I set would open up so much more room in my life.

Stepping away from my work at the residential facility broke my heart. It also opened up room for deeper healing and new skills that would bring me into my next season. I still get to serve those going through hard seasons and struggling with mental health issues; now, I get to do that through writing and speaking for a living.

Choosing to spend time apart on my visits to family opened up room for more joy, more laughter, and more connection with less frustration and stress. And learning to set healthy boundaries with myself has made room for so much more of what I want in life: more vision, more joy, more peace, more times my body feels good.

Of course, it makes perfect sense: weeds choke out flowers in a garden if they're left to grow unchecked. And if there aren't good fences, plants can easily get trampled. But when we set up boundaries, healthy things are allowed to grow and flourish without being overrun.

That's what your soul needs, friend—space to grow and flourish, to get stronger and healthier, more able to withstand the ups and downs of life.

Seventeen

Even If

Maybe it was a mistake to come here, I think. I'm not shaking hard enough that anyone would notice, but it might just be a matter of time. I try not to focus on the dizziness, the way I can't quite catch my breath, and the cramping muscles as I will myself not to shudder.

At least I asked for my decaf to go. I weigh my options and wait for my latte. *Should I bolt for the safety of my car? If I stay, am I going to get any work done or simply melt into tears?*

My face is a mask of calm but my gut is in knots. I want to stay and work. I slip the orange bottle from my purse and gulp down a tiny white tablet.

My face burns at the thought of someone seeing me take that pill, but I can't bring myself to look up to see if anyone did. I realize there's a million reasons someone could take prescription medication in a coffee shop, like blood pressure or migraines or diabetes. But part of me still shrinks and wants to cover the fact that I need something to soften the knots and gnarls inside me.

It's been like clockwork: anxiety attacks every afternoon.

I text Micah, tell him I'm struggling, then breathe deep and settle at my laptop. *It's going to be okay.* My heart rate smooths out and I start to feel a little sleepy.

But there's a sudden urgency in the tears burning the edges of my eyes. I'm thinking about how the meds will wear off in a few hours when I'm home with my husband. I hate that he isn't getting the best of me these days.

Shadrach, Meshach, and Abednego were Hebrew exiles in Babylon under the reign of Nebuchadnezzar. One day, the king decided to set up a huge golden statue and demand that everyone bow down to worship it. If anyone refused, he would be thrown into a fiery furnace and burned alive.

Nebuchadnezzar summoned all his officials and advisers to the dedication ceremony and told them to listen for the cue: an orchestra playing all kinds of music would tell them when to fall on their faces before the golden statue. Sure enough, it happened just like he commanded.

You probably know what comes next: Shadrach, Meshach, and Abednego refused to bow down. King Nebuchadnezzar gave them a second chance, taunted them, and asked what god could possibly rescue them from this peril. Again, they refused to bow.

> Shadrach, Meshach and Abednego replied to him, "King Nebuchadnezzar, we do not need to defend ourselves before you in this matter. If we are thrown into the blazing furnace, the God we serve is able to deliver us from it, and he will deliver us from Your Majesty's hand. But even if he does not, we want you to know, Your Majesty, that we will not serve your gods or worship the image of gold you have set up." (Daniel 3:16–18, NIV)

Of course, the king was furious. He had them tied up and tossed into the fiery furnace. The flames were so hot that they killed the soldiers who threw the exiles into the inferno. Nebuchadnezzar seemed satisfied, thinking this was the end of the story, until he noticed something strange: the three young men were walking around in the furnace, untied and apparently unharmed. And there was a fourth figure with them who looked "like an angel" or "like a son of the gods" (verse 25, GNT, ESV).

The story ended happily: Shadrach, Meshach, and Abednego were called out of the furnace and Nebuchadnezzar praised the Lord, saying nobody could save like their God. The young men were restored to honor in the king's court. And for those of us who learned this story on a flannelgraph or an episode of *Veggie Tales,* the message is clear: obey God, no matter what happens. The promise is just as obvious: when we are faithful to God, he will rescue us.

But this passage has much more to say than the sanitized Sunday school lessons of our childhoods. Because we often skip over this painful truth: *God didn't save them from the fire.*[1]

He didn't stop them from experiencing it. He didn't change the king's mind or fill him with compassion. Those three young men were full of faith that God was *able* to deliver them, but they had no idea if he would. Because, in their short lives, Shadrach, Meshach, and Abednego had already walked through all kinds of hell.

They'd survived the siege in Jerusalem, where they would have seen countless people die of sickness and starvation, only to be among the few captives taken alive and marched to Babylon. They were of royal blood, considered nobility, now disgraced and forced to serve the king who had destroyed everything they knew and loved. God hadn't saved them from any of that.

And when they were about to be thrown into the fire, there was no way to know if God would save them. But they did know, deep in their bones, that God had been *with them* through everything. And that simple confidence was enough to inspire two of the most powerful words in Scripture: *even if.*

In the deepest dark, despair asks Nebuchadnezzar's question with a hissing tongue: "What god can save you from this?"

But that's the wrong question. Because Shadrach, Meshach, and Abednego weren't saved from the fire. Instead, God met them *in the fire.* Many scholars believe that the "angel" who showed up in the furnace was actually the preincarnate Christ. In other words, it was Jesus himself. And though I've never stood in a literal furnace, I can relate to that *even if* experience.

The quiet assurance that gets me through is this: my God is able to save me, to heal me, to erase the pain and heartache in a moment. *But even if he doesn't,* I refuse to bow to despair. Even if I'm never fully delivered, I know that God is good and present in my pain.

Even if nothing changes. Even if I don't get out of this. Even if the flames are raging and there's no escape and I have no choice but to sit in the fire. Even if I never get better and the black dog of depression hounds me till the day I die, Christ himself is with me in the midst of the flames.

So I can stand in the raging inferno and not be destroyed.

That's enough for me.

———

It would be nice to leave you with a story of complete restoration. Maybe that's what you expected when you picked up this book. I hate to disappoint you. Really, I do, if only for selfish reasons. I'd sure love to tell you about how I found the key that unlocked all the mysteries of mental illness or that one day God finally showed up and healed me.

After all, most Christians are used to seeing stories of triumph and transformation look a certain way: God vanquishes the Enemy and everyone lives happily ever after. We're taught that the things of God are tidy and certain, black and white and easy to tie up in a bow. Good people are blessed. Bad people are punished.

But that's not the truth and beauty of the gospel. At best, it's a fairy tale. At worst, it's a sham sold by dishonest people looking to gain something. It's also not my lived experience. My guess is, if you've stuck with me this long, it's not yours either. And that's okay.

Because I can promise you this: though we have bleak and hard and anxious days, ours are still stories of triumph. Ours are still stories of transformation. And even though Shadrach, Meshach, and Abednego didn't have a single hair singed or their clothes smelling like smoke, they surely came out of the fire changed. And so do we.

Like those exiles, we walked through all kinds of heartache before coming to the furnace. Though we didn't always see him, God was with us through it all. We may not smell like smoke or be destroyed by flames, but we have the great faith to believe he's good and kind and present when he walks through fire with us instead of plucking us from it.

In the fire, we learn that hope can't rest solely on the *actions* of

God, on miraculous healings, or on answers to mysteries we can't comprehend. Instead, our hope rests on the *character* of a God who is love, who somehow brings beauty out of the ugliest ashes. We don't have to be healed, we don't have to be on the other side of it, to know he's good and he's transforming us—even in the furnace.

———

I raise my eyes to see the golden-hour sunlight. *Dark days don't last forever.* I whisper it to myself and my soul responds to the truth. *It's all going to be okay.* Spring is here and the sun is shining. It's bathing people in that perfect light that makes everything more beautiful.

I might be fighting off a panic attack in a coffee shop. I might be in the midst of a major depressive episode for the first time in three years. I might fight to get out of the house or even out of bed, but I know now what I didn't know for years:

Nothing's wrong with me.

I'm going to be just fine.

I am no less loved, no less worthy.

This will probably hurt like crazy, but it's going to pass.

I don't have to pretend or force myself to smile. I don't have to hide the hurt.

But it sure isn't going to run my life.

I know all of this—the brain fog, the apathy, migraines and stomach pains, god-awful numbness and the crushing weight—all of this is just an illness. They're all symptoms, not signs of weakness. I know the dark thoughts I didn't want to admit to Micah and my therapist don't come from me, but the disease.

I know how to speak kindly to myself now. I know when to press through and when to take a break—at least better than I used to. I know to not blame myself. I know to extend grace. I know at some point, it's all going to be okay again.

But the real truth, the thing that I tell myself over and over, is that it *is* okay. Right now. I'm okay. I'm better than okay.

Even with my illness, I'm convinced that life is beautiful. I've learned to see the countless gifts woven in the fabric of each day, to delight in what it means to live as the beloved of God.

Even when my skin burns and my head pounds and my heart feels dead, there's so much good in my life. Just writing that sentence made me smile, made my heart stir in my chest like some sleeping thing waking.

Today, I am anxious. I don't know what's going to happen with our finances. I don't know how long this depressive episode will last. I don't know if I'll have to change meds or increase the frequency of my therapy sessions.

But years of doing hard and deep inner work have taught me this: I am loved. I am wanted. I am never alone. I see it in that gorgeous sunlight. In the blossoming trees across the road and the funny little bird hopping around by the café tables. I taste it in my (decaf) coffee. I feel it in the warmth and wind of spring that remind me of resurrection, faithfully returning every year. So even if all the colors around me seem dull, I know I'm going to be okay.

I'm living proof of beauty from ashes. My life is rich and full, better than I ever could have hoped. It's not perfect by any means, but it's really good. I live in a city I love. I get to do something I enjoy for a living. And I'm married to an incredible man who loves me harder than anyone else but God himself.

I mentioned earlier that Jamie Tworkowski wrote about how we can choose to stay in this world because life has a way of surprising us.[2] My life has been full of surprises: Paris and youth pastoring and travel and Micah and friendships around the globe. My silly nieces who FaceTime me every few days. Writing and being able to share my story in a way that helps people. I didn't see any of it coming, and I would have missed every sweet moment if I'd taken my life anytime along the way.

But the biggest surprise of all has been discovering that I can struggle with depression and anxiety, even sometimes dark thoughts of suicide, and still have a life with God full of peace, contentment, and even joy. I'm surprised by the self-compassion he's taught me, by the kindness I've learned to extend not just to others, but to myself. I'm surprised when I look in the mirror and like what I see, when I don't beat myself up for the smallest mistake, and when I rest in the simple confidence that I am fully loved and fully accepted.

Bad days still come and sometimes bad weeks and months. I'm living them now. But in those bad times, I've learned to cling to the Lord come hell or high water. I press my face into his clothes and breathe in deep. When I'm terrified or my chest feels like that fiery furnace, I lean in to him and listen.

And much as I would love him to wave his magic wand and put my soul back together without cracks and scars, I am grateful. I *know* the Comforter because I have been comforted. I *know* a God who sees me and is present with me. That makes all the difference.

This is where I want to leave you, sweet friend. We've talked about tools and meds and self-care plans, doctors and therapy and showing up to do the hard work over and over again. But above all else, this is what you need to know:

You aren't alone. You can do this. There are beautiful surprises ahead. And God is with you. Even—especially—in the fire.

Benediction

By the time you hold it in your hands, this book will have been three years in the making. I'm supposed to be sending it off to my publisher, but I just can't let it go yet. I can't let this time together end without praying for you. It won't be the first time; I've tried to carry you in my heart all through this process, remembering the reason these words matter is because *you* matter, because you need to know you're not alone in your ache. But this is likely the first time you'll hear me pray for you.

You may not be familiar with the practice of benediction. In many faith traditions, there are a few moments at the end of the service when the pastor or priest speaks a blessing over the people. These good words are a final moment of reflection, a chance to seal what God has done in hearts and minds during their time together. One of the most famous benedictions comes from Numbers 6:24–26 (NLT): "May the LORD bless you and protect you. May the LORD smile on you and be gracious to you. May the LORD show you his favor and give you his peace." I love these words, and I pray them—and so much more—over you. So let's take just a few more moments, and allow me to leave you with a few words of blessing and love.

I pray you know how proud I am that you're still here. If you've ever been plagued by thoughts of suicide or self-harm, if you've ever wished you could go to sleep forever, it's a miracle you're still standing, still seeking a life that's more than what you've known. May you cling tightly to the simple belief that you can learn to live well despite mental illness, that quality of life isn't just about circumstances or a diagnosis but also the skills you develop along the journey.

May you find joy as you go, not because you try to force yourself to choose it, but because you learn to cultivate it in mundane moments and tiny, easily overlooked gifts. And I pray you discover those are the moments that make you glad to be alive, when you feel the warmth of fresh laundry from the dryer, the sun on your skin, or the embrace of a loved one.

May you learn to value yourself enough to set healthy boundaries, even with yourself, that allow you to tend the great gift that is your beautiful soul. I pray you fight for wholeness, be ruthless with self-care, and commit to the way of self-compassion. May you speak to yourself as to a much-beloved child, in gentle tones and kind words. And as you lean in to the process of acceptance, I pray you feel the layers of self-inflicted shame and judgment peel away.

My friend, I pray you would know, wherever you are, that people like me are cheering you on. You are not alone. When hope seems impossible, elusive, and forever out of reach, may you find the friends, colleagues, family members, and strangers on the internet who help you through those darkest moments. There is a great cloud of witnesses who believe better things for you when you can't believe them for yourself. And I pray you remember to borrow hope from us when yours is running thin.

May you find a faith community that tenderly welcomes your aching heart and exemplifies the compassion of Jesus to you. As you learn to walk this road, I pray you become a voice for hope, that you find the courage to speak up about your pain in ways that connect you with others and make them also feel seen.

And when people fail, as they inevitably will, may you find the courage to try again, and again, and again. May you always remember that we are all broken, we all need each other, and there are people who care deeply about your pain.

I pray you find a life-giving support team, no matter how long it takes. May you connect with kind, compassionate doctors and therapists to help you understand and support your brain and body. I pray that you receive with gratitude whatever provision God has for your well-being, even if it comes in a pill or on a counselor's couch.

May those who enter the sacred space of trauma and pain be tender and wise as they walk with you toward greater wholeness. I pray you have the courage to face the hidden things that are hard to acknowledge, to sit with the broken pieces in the compassionate presence of well-trained professionals. May you be surprised at the restoration that happens there. As you look back, I pray you'll be awed at how showing up and digging into the hard things leads to peace and healing you couldn't imagine.

May your faith grow deep and wide enough for your questions, anger, ache, and lament. May you find the freedom to be fully honest in the presence of a God who doesn't leave and doesn't lie.

I pray you will find new, guilt-free, life-giving ways to relate to Christ, knowing there is nothing wrong with you for suffering with a mental illness. As you remember that, even in the Bible, Jesus didn't miraculously heal everyone, may you know true faith is walking with him through the pain, not just being delivered from it. And as you find him present even in the pit of hell, I pray your relationship with God is healed.

May the voice of love be the loudest you hear. May you beat back the hissing lies and know that God is neither disappointed nor ashamed of you, and that the truest thing about you is that you are wildly beloved by the Creator of all good things.

Whether or not depression becomes a distant memory for you someday, may you be confident that you are not disqualified from the full, abundant life Jesus promised. May you come to know the tenderness and kindness of God in ways you've never imagined. I pray you know the Comforter by being comforted, and that you come to know the peace of God in the fires of anxiety. When all seems bleak and the color is drained from your world, I pray you know that even if the darkness will always be there, God with Us will always be there in the darkness.

Finally, beloved, as you learn to live with your limp, to walk a road you might not have chosen, these words bear repeating: I pray you know, deep in your bones, that you are not alone, that you are loved, and that you are worthy of everything it takes to get better.

In the name of the One who is always near to the brokenhearted, Amen.

Appendix A

HOW TO HELP DEPRESSED
AND SUICIDAL LOVED ONES

Someone you care about is hurting. Maybe you know he's struggling with depression and trying to fight off thoughts of suicide; maybe it's just a suspicion you have. You want to say the right things to help your loved one, but it seems overwhelming and scary. You just don't know what to say or how to respond, and perhaps you're afraid of causing more harm.

It's okay to be nervous and that this isn't easy. That just means you love this person and you want to get it right. There's good news, friend: it doesn't have to be complicated, even if it is uncomfortable to talk about depression, suicide, or self-harm. And you are not alone; God is with you as you come near to help your loved one bear this burden.

In fact, God has given us a beautiful, tender example of care for those who are depressed and suicidal, tucked away in the story of Elijah. In 1 Kings 19 (NIV), we see this prophet alone, overwhelmed, and desperate. He had to run for his life into the wilderness to escape death threats from the very leaders he had been called to turn back to God. He must have felt like an utter failure. "I have had enough, LORD," he prayed. "Take my life."

It would be easy to look at Elijah and think he had no reason to despair. He was well acquainted with the power of a miracle-working God—how could he turn around and wish for death? How could he believe he was alone when the Lord was so clearly present in his life? In moments like this, it's tempting to start by reminding those struggling of biblical truth, but that's not what we need when we're hopeless. And it's not what God did.

Instead, God got really practical. He fed Elijah, made sure he got some rest, and acknowledged the truth that must have felt crushing to the prophet: "the journey is too much for you" (1 Kings 19:7, NIV). Later, God sat with Elijah and just listened to the anguish of his heart without trying to fix it. He allowed Elijah to lament without correcting him. Without telling him to choose joy, read the Bible more, or stop being selfish. Instead, he came close to his precious child in the gentleness of a low whisper (verses 9–12).

We can learn from this ministry of presence the Lord offers us. As the body of Christ, it's our great honor to bear one another's burdens, and it's going to mean so much that you simply enter into your loved one's suffering in the same way Christ enters ours. Of course, there are times to remind our loved ones of what is good and true and lovely; God did eventually speak to the lies Elijah believed about being all alone, about his lost sense of purpose and direction. But first, he cared for Elijah's practical needs, acknowledged his ache, and listened to his brokenhearted cries.

Friend, let's take some pressure off: your hurting loved one doesn't need you to have answers or to handle this perfectly. Those of us who wrestle with mental illness usually just need to know a few things: that we're loved, we're not alone, and someone will walk with us through the shadows. If you're not sure how to say this or what to do, here are some simple phrases to get you started:

"I care about you and I'm sorry you're hurting."

- If somebody hasn't opened up, but it seems like something's wrong, try saying, "I've noticed it seems like you're having a hard time. I'm concerned about you and would love to help. What's going on?"
- "This must be terribly hard. I can't imagine what it's like."
- "I'm not disappointed in you. My heart hurts with you."
- "Would you like a hug?"

"Your pain and your story are important."

- "You are important to me and you are not a burden. My life is better because you're part of it."
- "What is making you feel this way? How long has it been going on?"

- "Tell me more about that."
- "I'm so grateful you shared this with me."

"You aren't alone."

- "Can I come hang out? Will you come to a movie with me?" Keep asking or inviting over and over, even if your loved one usually turns you down.
- "I'm proud of you for fighting! It must be really tough, but you're doing a good job."
- "How are you doing today? Do you want to talk?"
- "You're not a bad person for feeling this way. Lots of other people struggle too."
- "There's really good help and we can find it together."
- "It won't always be like this. It can get better."
- "I don't have answers, but I'll help you find them. There are doctors, therapists, and psychiatrists who can help."
- "Have you talked to a good doctor, counselor, or psychiatrist about this? Can I help you find one and make an appointment?"
- "Can I drive you to the appointment/go to the doctor with you/ help you pick up your prescription/meet you afterward?"

Those phrases can be so helpful, but you might want a little more insight on how and when to use them. Walking with somebody through mental illness can be a long process, so here are some important things to consider.

Know Your Limits

It's important to recognize your limits in supporting your loved one. Unless you are a licensed and trained therapist, doctor, or psychiatrist, you simply are not equipped to provide medical or psychological advice. I know you want to fix this for your loved one, but you can't.

That can actually be a very good thing. Knowing you can't solve this problem allows you to be who your loved one really needs you to be: a caring, trusted member of her support system. Whether you're a friend, family member, church leader, or colleague, the best support you can offer is loving, nonjudgmental care that encourages your loved one to get the professional help he needs.

It usually feels scary and overwhelming for someone to find help when he's struggling with mental illness, especially suicidal thoughts. Oftentimes, people don't get the professional support they need because they don't know where to start. Offer to make the appointments and go with him. Help him write out questions to ask. See chapters 5 and 13 for tips on finding and working with good therapists; chapter 12 offers assistance for working with doctors or psychiatrists regarding medication.

Remind him he's worth everything it takes to get better. Send encouraging text messages. Tell him you're proud of him for fighting. The best thing you can do is let your loved one know you care, you're with him, and that you want to walk with him as he discovers what it means to live well even with his pain. Your kindness, compassion, and support will go further than you can imagine.

Know Warning Signs

Sometimes, you're not sure if your loved one is struggling but your gut tells you something's wrong. Understanding warning signs of severe depression and suicide can help you know how to support her. I've shared a lot of the symptoms of depression and anxiety throughout this book: sleeping too much or not enough, nausea, fatigue, brain fog, headaches, and a racing heart are all common, but you may not know she's experiencing these things. Those of us wrestling with mental illness will often leave clues that we need help, even if we don't overtly ask for it.

For example, you might notice someone losing interest in things she once enjoyed, struggling to practice healthy self-care (perhaps she's no longer eating healthy amounts or her personal hygiene seems to go downhill a bit), or isolating from other people. Changes in mood can be a clue as well, but don't just look for sadness: anger or irritability are also common manifestations of depression and anxiety.[1]

We know that those enduring a crisis can be at greater risk for suicide. Divorce and other relational losses or problems, job loss or financial catastrophes, bullying, loss of freedom (going into a nursing home or jail, for example), or diagnosis of a serious illness can all make the future seem so bleak that it's not worth going on. Any great grief, like the death of a close loved one, can precipitate a suicidal crisis, and any exposure to suicide increases somebody's risk of attempting it herself.

A lot of these signs may seem obvious, but QPR Institute, a great resource for suicide prevention training, lists some less overt signs that somebody might be at risk for suicide. You might notice her "putting her affairs in order" by doing things like making a will, giving away prized possessions, or saying goodbyes as though she won't be around. Increased use of alcohol or drugs is a risk factor, including a relapse after a period of sobriety or recovery. Many people are intoxicated at the time of a suicide attempt, and a relapse can bring feelings of shame and hopelessness for somebody fighting an addiction. But one of the most surprising signs of suicide risk is an unexpected change in interest in God or the afterlife, like leaving a faith community or suddenly wanting to "get right with God." These could be signs somebody has either given up on faith or is preparing to "meet their maker."[2]

Sometimes, we'll make indirect comments about our pain, hopelessness, or exhaustion that hint at the depths of our struggles. Before I got help, I used to say things like "I hate my life" or "I wish I could go to sleep and never wake up." A dear friend genuinely believed his young family would be "better off without him." Hints that someone may not be around much longer, comments about being a burden, or saying she "always ruins things for others" can be signs as well.

Others make more direct comments, like "I want to kill myself" or "I've been thinking about ending my life." It's jarring when somebody says that, and we don't want to believe she's serious, but the best bet is to assume she is and that this may be the only time she comes to someone for help. I know that can feel like a lot of pressure, but remember, you just need to help your loved one find hope, feel loved, and get the help she needs. Your compassion, kindness, and lack of judgment will go a long way.

Have Tough Conversations

Be willing to ask tough questions, even when it's scary. It's always better to have the conversation than to wait and possibly regret it later. If you notice several of these risk factors and signs and you're worried, you can ask, "Are you thinking about suicide?" or "I know sometimes people wish they were dead when they're struggling. Are you having those thoughts?" That simple question could free your loved one to be honest and get the help he needs.

If you don't feel comfortable taking such a direct approach, you can warm up to it with indirect questions. QPR Institute suggests asking, "Do you ever wish you could go to sleep and never wake up?" Or this series of questions: "Have you been unhappy lately? Have you been *very* unhappy lately? Have you been so unhappy lately you've thought about ending your life?" Make sure to phrase the question in a way that he feels like he could answer yes without disappointing you. Avoid saying something like "You're not thinking of hurting yourself/doing something stupid/killing yourself, are you?" That communicates judgment and makes it harder for him to be honest.[3]

Be sure to listen well and leave plenty of space for him to talk. Know your loved one may have a hard time getting the words out and it might take a while. Do your best to make it feel safe for him to open up and know you can process your own emotions with somebody else at a later time. This might be a painful conversation for you, but try not to project that pain onto the person sharing with you by saying things like "How could you leave me like that?" or "Don't you care about what happens to me?" Don't give him any reason to clam up or feel embarrassed about talking to you.

After he talks, validate his pain and overwhelm, just as God did when he acknowledged to Elijah that the journey would be too much for him (1 Kings 19:7). This is a great place to use many of those phrases above, like "I'm so sorry you're hurting." Next, try to get your loved one to commit to getting help. If you know you're going to have this conversation, have some resources handy. If not, just ask if he'll come with you to get help and tell him you'll find the therapist or doctor if needed. Say you're willing to help him find solutions to the problems that make life feel unlivable. Remember, suicide is usually about solving a problem—escaping from unbearable circumstances or pain. Any hope that he can learn to manage or overcome those problems can help save a life.[4]

Remove Lethal Means

Finally, be willing to have tough conversations about limiting access to lethal means. In the suicide prevention world, "lethal means" is the term for any method somebody could use to end her life. Suicide attempts often happen in a moment of crisis, so making sure your loved one doesn't have access to lethal means during that crisis can be the difference between life and death.[5]

This is a difficult conversation to have for many reasons. It's scary to think about your loved one having access to a way to hurt herself, and it's incredibly uncomfortable to ask directly what she would use to attempt suicide. But this could save your loved one's life, so it's well worth it. If your loved one shares that she's considered using a particular method, do what it takes to remove it from the home or limit her access to it. While you're at it, see if there's anything else you can do to help her stay safe, like making sure lethal doses of medication (even over-the-counter meds like acetaminophen, ibuprofen, or antihistamines) or objects she may use to harm herself aren't available.

But this can also be a sensitive topic for political reasons as we discuss access to firearms. I know my readers come from across the political spectrum and have varying perspectives on gun ownership and (for U.S. citizens) the Second Amendment. Don't worry; I'm not diving into that here. Instead, let's focus on some facts and what you can do to help keep your loved one safe.

The simple truth is that those who attempt suicide with a gun are more likely to die than those who don't. About 85 percent of firearm-related suicide attempts end in death. This is a drastic contrast with the fact that many of the more widely used methods end in death less than 5 percent of the time.[6] While women attempt suicide much more frequently, the highest rate of completed suicides is among middle-aged white men, which also happens to be a group with especially high rates of access to guns.[7]

If you know or suspect your loved one has access to a gun and you have reason to believe he may be depressed, please talk to him. Start by asking the above questions about how he's feeling and whether he's had thoughts of hurting himself. Next, tell him you love him and want to make sure he stays safe, so you'd like to brainstorm some ideas to accomplish that. Again, this can be a sensitive topic, so make sure he knows your only goal is to help him stay safe, not to deprive him of rights.

Is there a friend or family member who could store the guns for a while? If your loved one has a locking gun safe, ask if he would allow you to hold on to the key for a while. You can also look into renting a storage space at a shooting range, gun shop, or even a local storage facility. Finally, some law enforcement departments offer temporary storage of firearms.[8] You'll want to check with your local department and make sure your loved one feels comfortable with this before pursuing this option.

Know This Is a Process

There's a common saying in the substance-abuse treatment world that relapse is part of recovery. While this isn't always the case, it can be true of mental health issues as well. It might seem like your loved one gets better and then starts to struggle again. You might have multiple tough conversations, get frantic late-night phone calls or texts when she's battling thoughts of suicide, or feel like she's not making progress. This is hard. And it's pretty normal.

Make sure to follow up after that initial conversation. Just let her know you're thinking about her and ask how she's doing. Say you care about her and you believe in her. Tell her you're proud of her for fighting and that she's doing a good job, like my pastor told me when I was struggling with self-harm. Those simple words are like oxygen to somebody battling suicidal thoughts or severe depression.

Don't neglect your own self-care. These are heavy things to help someone carry, so make sure you have somebody to talk to and process with. Make your own appointment with a counselor, or join a support group for family members of those with mental illness. Prioritize things that are refreshing and good for your soul. And if possible, help your loved one to build a support team so you don't feel like you have to carry her pain alone. This includes a good therapist and doctor, but also supportive friends, family members, a small group at church, or a support group. The more people she has in her corner, the more successful she will be and the easier it will be for you to walk with her for the long term.

When to Seek Emergency Help

If you think your loved one may hurt himself, please don't try to handle the situation without support. The National Suicide Prevention Lifeline is available 24/7 at 1-800-273-TALK (1-800-273-8255). You can also reach the Crisis Text Line by texting the word HOME to 741741. Trained volunteers can help you navigate the situation and come up with a plan of action. However, if you suspect your loved one is in immediate danger, do not leave him alone. Call 911 or take him to an emergency room (or an emergency mental health facility, if available in your area) if you can safely do so. Stay with him until he is safely in the care of a medical professional. In the moment, you may not be sure if you're doing the right thing, and your loved one might initially be upset. It's better to err on the side of lifesaving action and helping your loved one get professional support. You're doing the right thing, and your help could make all the difference in the world.

Appendix B

ADDITIONAL RESOURCES

Many of these resources have been immensely helpful on my mental health journey, while others are tools I wish I had when I was learning to manage my depression. While some come from a Christian perspective, others do not. All of them either provide valuable information or remind you you're not alone as you build a healthy life despite mental illness.

Mental Health and Suicide Prevention Resources

- National Suicide Prevention Lifeline—1-800-273-TALK (1-800-273-8255)
- Crisis Text Line—text the word HOME to 741741
  QPR Suicide Prevention Training—https://qprinstitute.com
- American Foundation for Suicide Prevention—https://afsp.org
- Find a counselor or therapist—www.psychologytoday.com/us/therapists

Books to Help You Feel Less Alone

- *If You Feel Too Much: Thoughts on Things Found and Lost and Hoped For* by Jamie Tworkowski
- *Reasons to Stay Alive* by Matt Haig (this book discusses suicidal thoughts in detail, so please use caution if that may be triggering for you)
- *Glorious Weakness: Discovering God in All We Lack* by Alia Joy (this book discusses suicidal thoughts/behavior in detail, so please use caution if that may be triggering for you)

- *This Too Shall Last: Finding Grace When Suffering Lingers* by K.J. Ramsey
- *Everything Happens for a Reason: And Other Lies I've Loved* by Kate Bowler

Books to Help You Understand How Your Brain and Body Work

- *The Body Keeps the Score: Brain, Mind, and Body in the Healing of Trauma* by Bessel van der Kolk
- *Try Softer: A Fresh Approach to Move Us out of Anxiety, Stress, and Survival Mode—and into a Life of Connection and Joy* by Aundi Kolber
- *Anatomy of the Soul: Surprising Connections Between Neuroscience and Spiritual Practices That Can Transform Your Life and Relationships* by Curt Thompson
- *How God Changes Your Brain: Breakthrough Findings from a Leading Neuroscientist* by Andrew Newberg
- *Mindsight: The New Science of Personal Transformation* by Daniel Siegel
- *The Mindful Way Through Depression: Freeing Yourself from Chronic Unhappiness* by Mark Williams, John Teasdale, Zindel Segal, and Jon Kabat-Zinn
- *The Inflamed Mind: A Radical New Approach to Depression* by Edward Bullmore

Books to Help You Connect with God Despite Pain

- *The Ragamuffin Gospel* and *The Furious Longing of God* by Brennan Manning
- *Embracing the Love of God: The Path and Promise of Christian Life* by James Bryan Smith
- *Miracles and Other Reasonable Things: A Story of Unlearning and Relearning God* by Sarah Bessey
- *One Thousand Gifts: A Dare to Live Fully Right Where You Are* and *The Broken Way: A Daring Path into the Abundant Life* by Ann Voskamp

Organizations, Podcasts, and People to Follow Online

- *CXMH* podcast hosted by Dr. Holly K. Oxhandler and Robert Vore, https://cxmhpodcast.com/
- *Faith & Mental Wellness* podcast hosted by Brittney Moses, https://brittneyamoses.com
- Fresh Hope for Mental Health, www.freshhope.us
- "Mental Health" on The Mighty, https://themighty.com/topic/mental-health
- Steve Austin, https://catchingyourbreath.com
- To Write Love on Her Arms, https://twloha.com

Acknowledgments

I've wept many tears over my laptop as I've tapped out these words. Sure, parts of my story have been painful to revisit, but most of those tears have come as I've thought of the many people who have loved and carried me—and this message—through the deepest anguish I've ever known. I am alive today because of some of you. I am healthy because of others. There are no words of gratitude that will ever suffice, so instead I'll ugly cry in this coffee shop and try my best to honor your care and contributions (and not forget anybody).

To the friends who have helped me get healthier, been safe places to land, and carried me through dark days, I owe you my life, my joy, and my wholeness. You believed in better things for me when I couldn't, you accepted my broken pieces, and you saw beauty where I saw only shame.

Cody and Jaina Hamilton, I still love Jesus because you showed me how to walk through hard things clinging to hope and how to lead with integrity even when it hurts. Thanks for believing in me, mentoring me, and loving me despite my stubbornness. Your faithfulness is awe inspiring.

Michael and Angela Pinkston, thank you for U2 and blackberry picking, folk festivals and teaching me to love coffee. Thanks for making me stay on your couch and telling me that God likes me. My long, slow walk toward wholeness started in your living room. Who knew it would turn into this?

Brooke and Ben Pitman, you're the real deal. Thanks for that summer in Panama City, taking me to camp, and amazing curry. I was scared and sad, but you loved me well. I'm so lucky to know you.

Kyle and Casey Wallace, you invited a newly unemployed stranger to your home, got me to move here, and sustained me with grilled cheese and soup during a hard season of transition. You were my first Nashville friends, and I'm living a beautiful life here because of you.

Steve and Lindsey Austin, you're my favorite former strangers from the internet. Thanks for helping me stay safe, telling me to get my butt in the car and start driving, for Frios and pool days and much-needed normalcy. Steve, so much of this book is because you showed up in a Facebook group you shouldn't have and told me I had a story to tell. Look how far we've come!

Alexis, Becca, Blake, Emily, Kate, Kelly, and all the other friends who walked with me through those dark days in Atlanta, you responded with such grace, even when you didn't know what to say or do. Thanks for pushing me, hoping when I couldn't, and sharing your own pain to remind me I wasn't alone.

To the wonderful people of my first church in Redmond, Oregon, thank you for welcoming me like a long-lost daughter. We were a young church, just trying to find our way, but I believe we were doing the best we could with what we had. I will always be grateful for the way you nourished my faith and believed in me.

To Cross Point, and especially Drew Powell, I breathed a sigh of relief when I heard you talk about mental illness from the stage. Thank you for being a safe community for people like me.

To Jenna and Megan, the therapists who taught me what it means to be seen, heard, and believed, professionals like you are the unsung heroes behind so much health and thriving in this world. I hope you see how your work ripples far beyond the clients on your couches. This book wouldn't exist without you.

To the incredible team that has brought this book into existence, you've made this process a joy. I feel like the luckiest author in the world to work with such professional, caring folks.

Tawny Johnson, I tear up every time I tell the story of you seeing that article on a friend's Facebook page and how you knew this was a book before I did. I was terrified and overwhelmed, but you waited months for me to make up my mind. You have taken such good care of me and I'm so grateful for you.

To all those at WaterBrook and Penguin Random House, thank you for bringing this book to life. Becky Nesbitt and Ashley Hong, your insight, care, and wisdom have made the editing process a delight. Thank you for challenging me, pushing me, and making me a better writer. Julia Wallace, Jennifer Backe, Laura Wright, and Sarah Horgan, thanks for turning these words into something tangible that people can hold close in their darkest moments. Lisa Beech, Jamie Lapeyrolerie, Ginia Hairston Croker, and Julie Smyth, thank you for helping me get this book to those in desperate need of hope.

Dr. Chinwe Williams, thank you for your wisdom and expertise as you reviewed the manuscript.

I'm so grateful for the many strangers on the internet who have championed this message, helped me figure out how to turn it into a book, and walked with me over the past several years.

Jeff Goins, you always say every story of success is a story of community. I'm glad you're part of mine. You've been a great mentor, and I'm grateful to call you friend. To my friends from Tribe Writers, Portfolio People Mastermind, and WAB, your belief in this message has sustained me in doubting seasons.

To Emily Freeman, Brian Dixon, Gary Moreland, and Myquillyn Smith, thank you for creating a community that models a gentle, soulful way to reach people. Special thanks to all my friends from Hope*Writers who have provided support, ideas, inspiration, encouragement, and feedback on subtitles and cover designs. I love running alongside you and watching your dreams materialize.

To the online faith and mental health community—Dr. Holly Oxhandler, Robert Vore, Brad Hoefs, Laura Howe, Brittney Moses, Aundi Kolber, K.J. Ramsey, and so many others—it's a joy to get to do this work with you. You give me courage to show up and share the hardest parts of my story. Thank you.

I owe a huge debt of gratitude to my early readers: Angela Hill, Claire G., Clark Roush, PhD, Grace North, Jake Kern, Jane W., Katie Moon, Katie R. Dale, L. A. Siewe, Michelle Krieg, Sara B., and others. Your comments, questions, and stories shaped this book immensely.

Special thanks to Alia Joy for early, generous help with my proposal and Andre Henry for publishing the original article that led to this book.

To the friends and family who asked, supported, and loved me through this process, you mean the world to me. Kristin, Amanda, Megan, Sam, Katee, Andrea, Sara, and Sherri, your friendship means so much to me. You've checked on me, prayed for me, laughed with me, and encouraged me more than I can say. Also, special thanks to Michelle Parker for lending me her house (and her very loud cat) to finish the manuscript. You are a treasure.

Erin and Ashley, I'd hide a body for you (but I'd rather not). You've both walked through hell and are building beautiful lives. It's an honor to call you friends.

To my sister, Leah, thanks for hacking my social media accounts to make me laugh, sending me the ridiculous things the girls say, and making me giggle harder than almost anybody else in the world. You say that sisters can't also be best friends, but I think you're wrong.

Mom and Dad, thanks for letting me read anything I could get my hands on. Few parents threaten to ground their kids from reading. I'm glad you never went through with it.

One of the greatest honors of my life has been to walk with those who have trusted me with their stories and pain. Whether I met you in a ministry, residential facility, or somewhere else, your vulnerability and courage have marked me; now, I see your faces when I write. It's been a joy to watch you stare down hard things, fight for wholeness, and live better stories than the ones you were handed. I'm immensely proud of you.

Micah, being married to you is the most fun I've ever had. You hold me through panic attacks, make sure I eat well, and champion my dreams. This book wouldn't have gotten written without your unending support. You're my very favorite and I post-holiday like you.

Finally, to Jesus, you're still everything to me. Sometimes, I still wish you would wave your magic wand and make me better, but I wouldn't trade the way I've gotten to know you for all the healing in the world. Thank you for the long road, for letting me scream and swear at you, and for proving over and over that you're Immanuel. You're the truest thing I've ever known.

Notes

Introduction: How to Use This Book

1. Jamie Tworkowski, founder of To Write Love on Her Arms, has written about this idea that life can surprise us, that when we're stuck in our pain we can forget that there are beauty and goodness ahead that we can't fathom. Check out Jamie's essays "And So We Hope to Be Surprised" at https://twloha.com/blog/and-so-we-hope-be-surprised and "There Is Still Some Time" at https://twloha.com/blog/there-still-some-time or in his book *If You Feel Too Much: Thoughts on Things Found and Lost and Hoped For* (New York: TarcherPerigee, 2016).

2. Carol S. Dweck, *Mindset: The New Psychology of Success* (New York: Ballantine, 2008), 6–7.

3. Dweck, *Mindset,* 38–39.

4. Dweck, *Mindset,* 38–39.

5. For more on how trauma impacts our mental health, see chapter 11 of this book.

6. God is much more than male; after all, he is spirit and doesn't possess a gendered body. Scripture is full of beautiful, feminine descriptions of God. In the original Hebrew for Genesis 1:1–2, God is referred to in both masculine and feminine terms as "Spirit" is a feminine noun. God is also described as giving birth (Deuteronomy 32:18; Isaiah 42:14; James 1:18, where the phrase "brought us forth" implies "from the womb" in the Greek), a nursing mother (Isaiah 49:15), a mother comforting her children (Isaiah 66:13), and even as a mother animal protecting her young (Deuteronomy 32:11–12; Psalm 17:8; Hosea 13:8; Matthew 23:37; and Luke 13:34).

Chapter One: Loving Jesus Doesn't Cure You

1. For more on the subtle influence of prosperity theology on our beliefs about healing, see Kate Bowler's excellent book *Everything Happens for a Reason: And Other Lies I've Loved* (New York: Random, 2018).

Chapter Two: People Say Terrible Things (But We Still Need Them)

1. Curt Thompson, *Anatomy of the Soul: Surprising Connections Between Neuroscience and Spiritual Practices That Can Transform Your Life and Relationships* (Carol Stream, IL: Tyndale, 2010), 111.

2. Thompson, *Anatomy of the Soul,* 111.

3. Annie G. Rogers, *A Shining Affliction: A Story of Harm and Healing in Psychotherapy* (New York: Viking, 1995), 256.

4. Siv Grav et al., "Association Between Social Support and Depression in the General Population: The HUNT Study, a Cross-Sectional Survey," *Journal of Clinical Nursing* 21, no. 1–2 (January 2012): 111–20, https://doi.org/10.1111/j.1365-2702.2011.03868.x.

5. Marilyn Baetz and John Toews, "Clinical Implications of Research on Religion, Spirituality, and Mental Health," *Canadian Journal of Psychiatry* 54, no. 5 (May 2009): 292–98, https://journals.sagepub.com/doi/pdf/10.1177/070674370905400503.

6. Harold G. Koenig, "Religion, Spirituality, and Health: The Research and Clinical Implications," *ISRN Psychiatry* 2012 (December 16, 2012), https://doi.org/10.5402/2012/278730.

7. Koenig, "Religion, Spirituality, and Health," 4.2.1, 4.3, 4.4.

Chapter Three: "I'm Not Disappointed in You"

1. Curt Thompson, *Anatomy of the Soul: Surprising Connections Between Neuroscience and Spiritual Practices That Can Transform Your Life and Relationships* (Carol Stream, IL: Tyndale, 2010), 192–95.

2. Daniel J. Siegel, *Mindsight: The New Science of Personal Transformation* (New York: Bantam, 2010), 195–96.

3. Aundi Kolber, *Try Softer: A Fresh Approach to Move Us out of Anxiety, Stress, and Survival Mode—and into a Life of Connection and Joy* (Carol Stream, IL: Tyndale Momentum, 2020), 166.

Chapter Four: Learning to Be Loved

1. Brother Lawrence, *The Practice of the Presence of God* (New Kensington, PA: Whitaker House, 1982).

2. Theophan the Recluse, quoted in Henri J. M. Nouwen, *The Way of the Heart: The Spirituality of the Desert Fathers and Mothers* (New York: HarperOne, 1981), 37–38, Kindle.

3. Henri J. M. Nouwen, *Life of the Beloved: Spiritual Living in a Secular World* (New York: Crossroad, 2002).

4. Curt Thompson, *Anatomy of the Soul: Surprising Connections Between Neuroscience and Spiritual Practices That Can Transform Your Life and Relationships* (Carol Stream, IL: Tyndale, 2010), 253.

5. Paul R. Albert, "Adult Neuroplasticity: A New 'Cure' for Major Depression?" *Journal of Psychiatry and Neuroscience* 44, no. 3 (2019): 147–50, https://doi.org/10.1503/jpn.190072.

6. Barbara Bradley Hagerty, "Prayer May Reshape Your Brain . . . and Your Reality," *All Things Considered,* NPR, May 20, 2009, www.npr.org/templates/story/story.php?storyId=104310443.

7. Andrew Newberg and Mark Robert Waldman, *How God Changes Your Brain:*

Breakthrough Findings from a Leading Neuroscientist (New York: Ballantine, 2009), 110–11.

8. Newberg and Waldman, *How God Changes Your Brain,* 56.

9. Brennan Manning, *The Furious Longing of God* (Colorado Springs: David C. Cook, 2009), 46.

10. Thompson, *Anatomy of the Soul,* 107.

11. Thompson, *Anatomy of the Soul,* 107.

Chapter Five: Bad Therapy

1. Oregon Revised Statutes. § 675.825(3)(b), www.oregonlaws.org/ors/675.825.

2. J. J. Lambert and D. E. Barley, "Research Summary on the Therapeutic Relationship and Psychotherapy Outcome," abstract, *Psychotherapy: Theory, Research, Practice, Training* 38, no. 4 (October 2001): 357–61, https://doi.org/10.1037/0033-3204.38.4.357.

3. Constantina Stamoulos et al., "Psychologists' Perceptions of the Importance of Common Factors in Psychotherapy for Successful Treatment Outcomes," *Journal of Psychotherapy Integration* 26, no. 3 (September 2016): 300–317, https://doi.org/10.1037/a0040426.

Chapter Six: Permission to Be Broken

1. "What About Pain?" Taking Charge of Your Health and Wellbeing, University of Minnesota, www.takingcharge.csh.umn.edu/explore-healing-practices/holistic-pregnancy-childbirth/what-about-pain.

2. Brett Q. Ford et al., "The Psychological Health Benefits of Accepting Negative Emotions and Thoughts: Laboratory, Diary, and Longitudinal Evidence," *Journal of Personality and Social Psychology* 115, no. 6 (December 2018): 1075–92, https://doi.org/10.1037/pspp0000157.

3. Lauren Mizock, "Five Tips to Accept a Mental Health Problem," *Psychology Today,* February 27, 2017, www.psychologytoday.com/us/blog/the-health-women/201702/five-tips-accept-mental-health-problem.

4. Bessel van der Kolk, *The Body Keeps the Score: Brain, Mind, and Body in the Healing of Trauma* (New York: Penguin, 2014), 97.

5. Mark Williams et al., *The Mindful Way Through Depression: Freeing Yourself from Chronic Unhappiness* (New York: Guilford, 2007), 35.

6. Williams et al., *Mindful Way Through Depression,* 36.

7. I first heard this illustration in relationship to addiction research and ACT therapy in Jonathan Bricker, "The Secret to Self-Control," 15:13, December 22, 2014, TEDx video, YouTube, www.youtube.com/watch?v=tTb3d5cjSFI.

Chapter Seven: Relapse, Reputation, and Risk

1. "Mental Health By the Numbers," National Alliance on Mental Illness, www.nami.org/mhstats.

2. For more on this topic, *Safe People* by Henry Cloud and John Townsend is a

great resource that discusses recognizing healthy and safe people to build relationships with. It also looks at why some of us are attracted to unsafe people and how to change that. The points in this section are taken from chapters 2 and 3 of this book.

3. This popular phrase has been attributed to Nadia Bolz-Weber, quoted in Michelle Gifford, "Share Your Story, Grow Your Business," *The Blog,* Michelle Gifford Creative, May 26, 2020, https://iammichellegifford.com/share-your-story-grow-your-business.

Chapter Eight: If I Make My Bed in Hell

1. Curt Thompson, *Anatomy of the Soul: Surprising Connections Between Neuroscience and Spiritual Practices That Can Transform Your Life and Relationships* (Carol Stream, IL: Tyndale, 2010), 65–68.

2. James Cartreine, "More than Sad: Depression Affects Your Ability to Think," *Harvard Health* (blog), Harvard Health Publishing, May 6, 2016, www.health.harvard.edu/blog/sad-depression-affects-ability-think-201605069551.

3. Thompson, *Anatomy of the Soul,* 150.

4. Wayne Cordeiro, "SOAP Study with Pastor Cordeiro," *Olive Tree* (blog), www.olivetree.com/blog/soap-cordeiro.

5. My friend Rev. Imani Ackerman has a very helpful guide here: "Why the SOAP Bible Study Isn't Enough (and What to Do Instead)," August 18, 2018, imaniackerman.com/soap-bible-study-ideas. Additional resources are www.blueletterbible.org, www.biblehub.com, www.biblegateway.com, and *Misreading Scripture with Western Eyes: Removing Cultural Blinders to Better Understand the Bible* by E. Randolph Richards and Brandon J. O'Brien.

Chapter Nine: The Darkness May Always Be There

1. "Mental Health Facts in America," National Alliance on Mental Illness, www.nami.org/nami/media/nami-media/infographics/generalmhfacts.pdf.

2. American Psychiatric Association, *Diagnostic and Statistical Manual of Mental Disorders,* 5th ed. (Arlington, VA: American Psychiatric Association, 2013), DSM-V. The relevant information is on pages 155, 166 (under "Course Modifiers"), 168 (under "Comorbidity"), and 171 (also under "Comorbidity") of the book.

3. Stephanie L. Burcusa and William G. Iacono, "Risk for Recurrence in Depression," *Clinical Psychology Review* 27, no. 8 (December 2007): 959–85, https://doi.org/10.1016/j.cpr.2007.02.005.

4. Kang Sim et al., "Prevention of Relapse and Recurrence in Adults with Major Depressive Disorder: Systematic Review and Meta-Analyses of Controlled Trials," *The International Journal of Neuropsychopharmacology* 19, no. 2 (July 2016), introduction, https://doi.org/10.1093/ijnp/pyv076.

5. World Health Organization, "U.S. Leading Categories of Diseases/Disorders," National Institute of Mental Health, www.nimh.nih.gov/health/statistics/disability/us-leading-categories-of-diseases-disorders.shtml.

6. Paul E. Greenberg et al., "The Economic Burden of Adults with Major Depressive Disorder in the United States (2005 and 2010)," *Journal of Clinical Psychiatry* 76, no. 2 (February 2015): 155–62, www.psychiatrist.com/jcp/article/pages/2015/v76n02/v76n0204.aspx.

Chapter Ten: Living with a Limp

1. "H3201–*yakol*–Strong's Hebrew Lexicon (KJV)," Blue Letter Bible, www.blueletterbible.org/lang/lexicon/lexicon.cfm?Strongs=H3201&t=KJV.

2. Daniel G. Amen, *The End of Mental Illness: How Neuroscience Is Transforming Psychiatry and Helping Prevent or Reverse Mood and Anxiety Disorders, ADHD, Addictions, PTSD, Psychosis, Personality Disorders, and More* (Carol Stream, IL: Tyndale, 2020), 89.

3. Amen, *End of Mental Illness,* 243.

4. Amen, *End of Mental Illness,* 244.

5. "Men and Mental Health," National Institute of Mental Health, www.nimh.nih.gov/health/topics/men-and-mental-health/index.shtml.

6. Substance Abuse and Mental Health Services Administration, "Racial/Ethnic Differences in Mental Health Service Use Among Adults," HHS Publication No. SMA-15-4906 (Rockville, MD: Substance Abuse and Mental Health Services Administration, 2015), www.samhsa.gov/data/report/racialethnic-differences-mental-health-service-use-among-adults.

7. Julie Corliss, "Mindfulness Meditation May Ease Anxiety, Mental Stress," *Harvard Health* (blog), Harvard Health Publishing, January 8, 2014, www.health.harvard.edu/blog/mindfulness-meditation-may-ease-anxiety-mental-stress-201401086967.

8. Leonard J. Hoenig, "Jacob's Limp," *Seminars in Arthritis and Rheumatism* 26, no. 4 (February 1997): 684–88, https://doi.org/10.1016/s0049-0172(97)80004-2.

Chapter Eleven: Sit in the Dark

1. The phrase "slowly then all at once" has been attributed to several authors including Mark Twain, F. Scott Fitzgerald, and a variation by Ernest Hemingway; it was more recently used by John Green in *The Fault in Our Stars.*

2. "H7503–*raphah*–Strong's Hebrew Lexicon (KJV)," Blue Letter Bible, www.blueletterbible.org/lang/lexicon/lexicon.cfm?Strongs=H7503&t=KJV.

3. While 2 Kings 24–25 and 2 Chronicles 36 record Jerusalem's destruction, the book of Lamentations paints a fuller and more brutal picture of the siege as well as the prophet Jeremiah's intense grief.

4. "What Causes Depression?" Harvard Health Publishing, June 24, 2019, www.health.harvard.edu/mind-and-mood/what-causes-depression.

5. Alexa Negele et al., "Childhood Trauma and Its Relation to Chronic Depression in Adulthood," *Depression Research and Treatment* 2015 (2015), https://doi.org/10.1155/2015/650804.

6. "Past Trauma May Haunt Your Future Health," Harvard Health Publishing, February 2019, www.health.harvard.edu/diseases-and-conditions/past-trauma-may-haunt-your-future-health.

Chapter Twelve: When Provision Comes in a Pill

1. "Treatment of Major Depressive Episode Among Adults" and "Prevalence of Major Depressive Episode Among Adolescents," Major Depression, National Institute of Mental Health, February 2019, www.nimh.nih.gov/health/statistics/major-depression.shtml.

2. "Suicide Rising Across the U.S.," *CDC Vital Signs*, Centers for Disease Control and Prevention, June 7, 2018, www.cdc.gov/vitalsigns/suicide/index.html.

3. Sarah Keller et al., "A Look at Culture and Stigma of Suicide: Textual Analysis of Community Theatre Performances," *International Journal of Environmental Research and Public Health* 16, no. 3 (January 26, 2019): 352, https://doi.org/10.3390/ijerph16030352.

4. Virginia K. Carroll, "Is a Medical Illness Causing Your Patient's Depression?" *Current Psychiatry* 8, no. 8 (August 2009): 43–54, www.mdedge.com/psychiatry/article/63655/medical-illness-causing-your-patients-depression.

5. Richard Nahas and Osmaan Sheikh, "Complementary and Alternative Medicine for the Treatment of Major Depressive Disorder," *Canadian Family Physician* 57, no. 6 (June 2011): 659–63, www.ncbi.nlm.nih.gov/pmc/articles/PMC3114664.

6. Marlene P. Freeman et al., "Complementary and Alternative Medicine in Major Depressive Disorder: The American Psychiatric Association Task Force Report," *Journal of Clinical Psychiatry* 71, no. 6 (2010): 669–81, https://doi.org/10.4088/JCP.10cs05959blu.

7. Felice N. Jacka et al., "A Randomised Controlled Trial of Dietary Improvement for Adults with Major Depression (the 'SMILES' Trial)," *BMC Medicine* 15 (2017), https://doi.org/10.1186/s12916-017-0791-y.

8. Chieh-Hsin Lee and Fabrizio Giuliani, "The Role of Inflammation in Depression and Fatigue," *Frontiers in Immunology* 10 (July 19, 2019), https://doi.org/10.3389/fimmu.2019.01696.

9. Daniel J. Siegel, *Mindsight: The New Science of Personal Transformation* (New York: Bantam, 2010), 83.

10. Sarah Boseley, "The Drugs Do Work: Antidepressants Are Effective, Study Shows," *The Guardian*, February 21, 2018, www.theguardian.com/science/2018/feb/21/the-drugs-do-work-antidepressants-are-effective-study-shows.

11. "Depression: How Effective Are Antidepressants?" Institute for Quality and Efficiency in Health Care, InformedHealth.org, June 18, 2020, www.ncbi.nlm.nih.gov/books/NBK361016.

12. Seth J. Gillihan, "What Is the Best Way to Treat Depression?" *Psychology Today*, May 30, 2017, www.psychologytoday.com/us/blog/think-act-be/201705/what-is-the-best-way-treat-depression.

13. Thomas Insel, "Antidepressants: A Complicated Picture," National Institute of Mental Health, December 6, 2011, www.nimh.nih.gov/about/directors/thomas-insel/blog/2011/antidepressants-a-complicated-picture.shtml.

14. Khalid Saad Al-Harbi, "Treatment-Resistant Depression: Therapeutic Trends, Challenges, and Future Directions," *Patient Preference and Adherence* 6 (2012): 369–88, https://doi.org/10.2147/PPA.S29716.

15. Jack Alan McCain, "Antidepressants and Suicide in Adolescents and Adults: A Public Health Experiment with Unintended Consequences?" *Pharmacy and Therapeutics* 34, no. 7 (2009): 355–67, 378, www.ncbi.nlm.nih.gov/pmc/articles/PMC2799109.

16. Matthew Gabriel and Verinder Sharma, "Antidepressant Discontinuation Syndrome," *Canadian Medical Association Journal* 189, no. 21 (May 29, 2017): E747, https://doi.org/10.1503/cmaj.160991.

17. Curt Thompson, *Anatomy of the Soul: Surprising Connections Between Neuroscience and Spiritual Practices That Can Transform Your Life and Relationships* (Carol Stream, IL: Tyndale, 2010), 252.

Chapter Thirteen: Good Therapy and Doing the Work

1. Curt Thompson, *Anatomy of the Soul: Surprising Connections Between Neuroscience and Spiritual Practices That Can Transform Your Life and Relationships* (Carol Stream, IL: Tyndale, 2010), 253.

2. Thompson, *Anatomy of the Soul,* 253.

3. Alex Korb, *The Upward Spiral: Using Neuroscience to Reverse the Course of Depression, One Small Change at a Time* (Oakland, CA: New Harbinger, 2015), 179.

4. Korb, *The Upward Spiral,* 179–86.

5. Edward Bullmore, *The Inflamed Mind: A Radical New Approach to Depression* (New York: Picador, 2018), 83.

6. Annie G. Rogers, *A Shining Affliction: A Story of Harm and Healing in Psychotherapy* (New York: Penguin, 1995), 256.

7. Kang Sim et al., "Prevention of Relapse and Recurrence in Adults with Major Depressive Disorder: Systematic Review and Meta-Analyses of Controlled Trials," *International Journal of Neuropsychopharmacology* 19, no. 2 (February 2016), https://doi.org/10.1093/ijnp/pyv076.

8. Kendra Cherry, "What Is Cognitive Behavioral Therapy (CBT)?" Verywell Mind, updated June 13, 2020, www.verywellmind.com/what-is-cognitive-behavior-therapy-2795747.

9. "Dialectical Behavior Therapy," Suicide Prevention Resource Center, 2006, www.sprc.org/resources-programs/dialectical-behavior-therapy.

10. For an in-depth look at how trauma impacts us—and how to heal from it—I highly recommend *Try Softer* by Aundi Kolber and *The Body Keeps the Score* by Bessel van der Kolk.

Chapter Fourteen: Beating Back the Darkness

1. "G25–*agapaō*–Strong's Greek Lexicon (KJV)," Blue Letter Bible, www.blueletterbible.org/lang/lexicon/lexicon.cfm?Strongs=G25&t=KJV.

2. "The Power of Self-Compassion," Harvard Health Publishing, www.health.harvard.edu/healthbeat/the-power-of-self-compassion.

3. Kristin Neff, "The Chemicals of Care: How Self-Compassion Manifests in Our Bodies," *Huffington Post,* June 27, 2011 www.huffpost.com/entry/self-compassion_b_884665?utm_campaign=share_email&ncid=other_email_o63gt2jcad4.

4. Aundi Kolber, *Try Softer: A Fresh Approach to Move Us out of Anxiety, Stress, and Survival Mode—and into a Life of Connection and Joy* (Carol Stream, IL: Tyndale Momentum, 2020), 192–95.

5. Martin Luther, Quotes, Goodreads, www.goodreads.com/quotes/757798-you -cannot-keep-birds-from-flying-over-your-head-but.

6. "KJV Search Results for *Joy*," Blue Letter Bible, www.blueletterbible.org/search/ search.cfm?Criteria=joy&t=KJV&lexicSt=2#s_lexiconc.

Chapter Fifteen: Ruthless with Self-Care

1. Sarah Bessey, *Miracles and Other Reasonable Things: A Story of Unlearning and Relearning God* (New York: Simon & Schuster, 2019), 169.

2. Aundi Kolber, *Try Softer: A Fresh Approach to Move Us out of Anxiety, Stress, and Survival Mode—and into a Life of Connection and Joy* (Carol Stream, IL: Tyndale Momentum, 2020), 67, 237.

3. Edward Bullmore, *The Inflamed Mind: A Radical New Approach to Depression* (New York: Picador, 2018), 19.

4. Bullmore, *Inflamed Mind*, 13–15.

5. Xueping Liu et al., "Genetic Factors Underlying the Bidirectional Relationship Between Autoimmune and Mental Disorders—Findings from a Danish Population-Based Study," *Brain, Behavior, and Immunity* (June 11, 2020), https:// doi.org/10.1016/j.bbi.2020.06.014.

6. Bullmore, *Inflamed Mind*, 176–78.

7. Bullmore, *Inflamed Mind*, 196.

8. Alex Korb, *The Upward Spiral: Using Neuroscience to Reverse the Course of Depression, One Small Change at a Time* (Oakland, CA: New Harbinger, 2015), 181.

9. Sam Manger, "Lifestyle Interventions for Mental Health" *Australian Journal of General Practice* 48, no. 10 (October 2019), www1.racgp.org.au/ajgp/2019/october/ lifestyle-interventions-for-mental-health.

10. Felice N. Jacka et al., "A Randomised Controlled Trial of Dietary Improvement for Adults with Major Depression (the 'SMILES' Trial)," *BMC Medicine* 15 (2017), https://doi.org/10.1186/s12916-017-0791-y.

11. Stephen S. Ilardi, *The Depression Cure: The Six-Step Program to Beat Depression* (Cambridge, MA: Da Capo, 2009), 13–15.

12. Ilardi, *Depression Cure*, 117.

13. Ilardi, *Depression Cure*, 121–22.

14. Kolber, *Try Softer*, 158–59.

15. Bessel van der Kolk, *The Body Keeps the Score: Brain, Mind, and Body in the Healing of Trauma* (New York: Penguin, 2014), 98–99, 164–65.

16. Curt Thompson, *Anatomy of the Soul: Surprising Connections Between Neuroscience and Spiritual Practices That Can Transform Your Life and Relationships* (Carol Stream, IL: Tyndale, 2010), 65–69.

17. Van der Kolk, *The Body Keeps the Score*, 91, 94–95.

18. Van der Kolk, *The Body Keeps the Score*, 103.

19. Van der Kolk, *The Body Keeps the Score*, 271–72.

20. Van der Kolk, *The Body Keeps the Score*, 275.

21. "Hobbies May Help Defeating Depression," *Journal of Psychotherapy and Psychosomatics*, Medical Press, May 25, 2020, https://medicalxpress.com/news/2020-05-hobbies-defeating-depression.html.

22. Alexander J. Scott, Thomas L. Webb, and Georgina Rowse, "Does Improving Sleep Lead to Better Mental Health? A Protocol for a Meta-Analytic Review of Randomised Controlled Trials," *BMJ Open* 7 (September 18, 2017), https://doi.org/10.1136/bmjopen-2017-016873.

23. "Sleep and Mental Health," *Harvard Mental Health Letter,* Harvard Health Publishing, March 18, 2019, www.health.harvard.edu/newsletter_article/sleep-and-mental-health.

24. "Sleep and Mental Health," Harvard Health Publishing.

Chapter Sixteen: Boundaries, Loving Others, and Soul-Keeping

1. Henry Cloud and John Townsend, *Boundaries: When to Say Yes, How to Say No to Take Control of Your Life* (Grand Rapids, MI: Zondervan, 2017), 30.

2. Aundi Kolber, *Try Softer: A Fresh Approach to Move Us out of Anxiety, Stress, and Survival Mode—and into a Life of Connection and Joy* (Carol Stream, IL: Tyndale Momentum, 2020), 93.

3. Kolber, *Try Softer,* 98.

4. Mary Oliver, "The Summer Day," *New and Selected Poems* (Boston: Beacon, 1992), 94.

Chapter Seventeen: Even If

1. Tim Mackie, "The National Idol—Faithfulness in Exile [Daniel]," BibleProject, YouTube video, 51:15, August 19, 2017, www.youtube.com/watch?v=3ja7S9Og4lA.

2. Jamie Tworkowski, *If You Feel Too Much: Thoughts on Things Found and Lost and Hoped For* (New York: TarcherPerigee, 2016), 161.

Appendix A: How to Help Depressed and Suicidal Loved Ones

1. "Risk Factors and Warning Signs," American Foundation for Suicide Prevention, https://afsp.org/risk-factors-and-warning-signs.

2. Paul G. Quinnett, *Suicide: The Forever Decision* (Chestnut Ridge: NY: Crossroad, 1992), QPR Gatekeeper Training, QPR Institute, https://qprinstitute.com/individual-training.

3. Quinnett, *Suicide,* QPR Gatekeeper Training.

4. Quinnett, *Suicide,* QPR Gatekeeper Training.

5. "Means Matter," Harvard School of Public Health, www.hsph.harvard.edu/means-matter.

6. "Means Matter: Firearm Access Is a Risk Factor for Suicide," Harvard School of Public Health, www.hsph.harvard.edu/means-matter/means-matter/risk.

7. "Suicide Statistics," American Foundation for Suicide Prevention, https://afsp.org/suicide-statistics.

8. "Means Matter: Families," Harvard School of Public Health, www.hsph.harvard.edu/means-matter/recommendations/families.

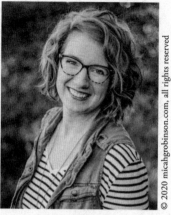

SARAH J. ROBINSON once believed her lifelong battle with depression made her a bad Christian. Now she's an author and speaker who helps others discover that mental illness doesn't disqualify them from living rich, beautiful lives in Christ. Drawing from a decade of ministry experience and the mental health field, Sarah helps readers fight for wholeness and cultivate joy at sarahjrobinson.com. She lives in Nashville with her husband.